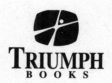

TRIUMPH
B O O K S

EDDIE OLCZYK
BEATING THE ODDS IN HOCKEY AND IN LIFE

Eddie Olczyk
with Perry Lefko

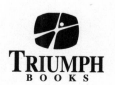

TRIUMPH
BOOKS

Library of Congress Cataloguing-in-Publication Data available upon request

This book is available in quantity at special discounts for your group or organization. For further information, contact:

Triumph Books LLC
814 North Franklin Street
Chicago, Illinois 60610
(312) 337-0747
www.triumphbooks.com

Printed in U.S.A.
ISBN: 978-1-62937-841-1
Design by Patricia Frey
Photos courtesy of Eddie Olczyk unless otherwise indicated

My ultimate purpose with this book is to try to inspire as many people as I can who are making life-altering decisions and choices and facing obstacles at every turn. If I can make one person laugh, cry, or love or believe more in themselves or someone else, I have scored the most important goal of my life.

—E.O.

To my wife, Jane, who is the Hall of Famer in the Lefko family, and our great children, Ben and Shayna. Their belief in me is what makes me write books and tell stories. Words matter!

—P.L.

CONTENTS

FOREWORD *by Pat Foley*   ix

INTRODUCTION   xiii

CHAPTER 1.   The Call   1

CHAPTER 2.   The Birth of a Rink Rat   15

CHAPTER 3.   The Olympics   27

CHAPTER 4.   Coming Home   39

CHAPTER 5.   Eddie Olczyk, Chicago Blackhawk   47

CHAPTER 6.   Heading North   59

CHAPTER 7.   Life as a Leaf   65

CHAPTER 8.   A Question of Timing   89

CHAPTER 9.   No More 1940   109

CHAPTER 10.   Good-bye, New York; Hello,
              Winnipeg (Again)   133

CHAPTER 11.   From L.A. to the Burgh   141

CHAPTER 12.   Farewell, Hockey   153

CHAPTER 13.   A New Perspective   159

CHAPTER 14.   Behind the Bench, Briefly   167

CHAPTER 15.   Back to the Booth   189

CHAPTER 16.   The Calls to the Halls   209

CHAPTER 17.   Witnessing History   217

CHAPTER 18.   Going 12 Rounds with Cancer   227

CHAPTER 19.   Getting Back on the Broadcasting Horse   255

CHAPTER 20.   A Blessed Union   265

CHAPTER 21.   One More Shift   269

CHAPTER 22.   A Rangers Reunion   275

CHAPTER 23.   Witnessing History (Again)   279

CHAPTER 24.   Thank God I Got Sick   287

AFTERWORD   293

ACKNOWLEDGMENTS   315

FOREWORD

YOUR LIFE IS PERFECT. You're 51 years old. You married the love of your life. You and Diana raised four outstanding kids. You were drafted third overall by the Chicago Blackhawks, the team you cheered for as a child. You played the first and last game of a terrific 1,000-plus-game career for them, a career that put you in the U.S. Hockey Hall of Fame. You have a broadcasting career that has you working for your favorite team, and that evolved into you becoming an award-winning network analyst. Not just for one sport but two, hockey and your other love, horse racing. You are the only person on television who can say that. Perfect.

Then all of a sudden, your world is shaken. Your future is in doubt. Stage 3 colon cancer.

What does somebody do when a friend has a bomb like that dropped in their lap? All I could think was, be there for Eddie. Be a friend, be supportive, be uplifting. So when I called him every day, I had one goal: I tried to get him laughing because he was as down as anybody could be. Anything to get his mind off his sickness for even a minute. About three weeks into the process I realized I was out of bullets and that I'd told him every joke I've ever heard. So I just found a way to tell him something goofy that happened on the plane or that somebody said.

There were all these people around the National Hockey League asking about him. It was quite remarkable to witness and be a conduit for the amount of concern and love he generated around the league. I told them all, "Call him, he's got time." Those calls really helped him, and they happened because people had found out what I had known since 1984: he's a good guy.

When he was diagnosed with colon cancer, he chose to go public with it. Many would have wanted to fight that battle privately, but he felt he could help people by raising awareness—and he did. I got a colonoscopy and I know many Blackhawks employees who did the same. Did Eddie Olczyk save lives? I believe that case could be made. God bless him.

He's always had an open and welcoming soul. But now having dealt with what he did, he is a huge help to people and families who are dealing with cancer. I've seen many interactions where people leave Eddie's company with hope. That's huge.

I think Eddie is the best analyst in all of sports. I've always said he has a photographic memory. His ability to dissect and immediately break down plays is remarkable. It's one of his many gifts as a broadcaster. He and I look at broadcasting Blackhawks games the same way: we hope to be instructional and we hope to be entertaining. He's got a great sense of humor, we both like to laugh, and that's always been a part of what we do. You can't manufacture that. We've had chemistry since the first time I sat next to him. We both want to do our jobs well and all of that, but we're in the entertainment business. We want Blackhawks broadcasts to be fun, something to look forward to, and that's what we're aiming for.

Many viewers seemed surprised when we expressed our love for each other on the air during his illness. It was probably a little bit deeper than a lot of broadcast partners would be, but that's how I feel about him. It's wonderful to sit next to a guy who is great at his job and is a great friend. He can trust me and I can trust him. We're both all in, so it's really awesome.

You know the one thing that's changed since he went through his battle? We hug more now. That's cool.

Enjoy this amazing story. And don't forget, Eddie Olczyk saved lives.

Pat Foley is entering his 37th season as the play-by-play voice of the Chicago Blackhawks. In 2014, he was selected as the Hockey Hall of Fame Foster Hewitt Memorial Award winner for outstanding contributions as a hockey broadcaster. Foley partners with Eddie Olczyk to broadcast all Blackhawks games on NBC Sports Chicago and WGN-TV Channel 9.

INTRODUCTION

WE'VE ALL BEEN THROUGH challenges in our lives. When I was growing up—say, between the ages of eight and 16—friends, teammates, their parents, and some coaches told me I'd never make it into the National Hockey League. They pointed out that most NHL players born in the 1960s were Canadians, and that few of the Americans who did break through were from Chicago, like I was.

When I was trying out for the U.S. Olympic team as a 16-year-old back in 1983, people told me I'd never make it because I was too young.

After I made it to the NHL, some people told me I'd eat my way out of the league. What's wrong with a hungry hockey player? Nothing like a well-done end-cut piece of prime rib, by the way.

People told me I could never be the first American-born lead hockey analyst on national TV in the U.S.

I proved all of those people wrong.

But I did not have one person tell me that I would lose my battle with cancer. Everybody told me I was going to beat this thing, and that was the greatest support I've had and something that will stay with me for the rest of my life.

I know there are a lot of people with cancer who are much worse off than I am. I want to help them fight or inspire them when they are battling through the treatments, or keep a person away from this disease by reading my story and getting themselves checked out.

After my diagnosis, I asked my oncologist, "So you're telling me I am signing up for six months of hell with chemo in exchange for 50 more years on this earth?"

"That's the plan," she said.

"Okay, where do I sign? Let's go!"

EDDIE OLCZYK
BEATING THE ODDS IN HOCKEY AND IN LIFE

CHAPTER 1

THE CALL

THE HOME PHONE RANG at precisely 7:07 PM on August 4, 2017, and immediately I began to worry.

Because the phone is connected to the TV I was watching, I knew the call was from Northwestern Memorial Hospital. I also knew it couldn't be a good thing to be getting a call on a Friday night from the hospital four days after I had come home from surgery to remove a tumor from my colon.

I was still in bed recovering and my wife, Diana, asked me if I planned to answer the phone. I told her I knew it was Dr. Scott Strong, who had performed the surgery, and that he was probably calling with the results of the biopsy.

Diana answered the phone after five or six rings and then handed it over to me.

"Eddie, it's Dr. Strong," he said.

"Hey, Doc," I said.

"You have Stage 3 colon cancer and we're recommending six months of chemotherapy."

My first thought was, how long do I have to live?

I knew cancer has four stages, from one to four, with four being the most severe. I was 51 years old, married to Diana for 28 years and 363 days, and we were the proud parents of four wonderful children—Eddie, Tommy, Alexandra, and Nicholas.

How much longer would I live to see them? How do I tell them, my folks, my two brothers, friends, and the entire hockey world that I have Stage 3 colon cancer?

Dr. Strong said I needed to recover for about a month before beginning chemotherapy and that oncologist Dr. Mary Mulcahy would soon be in touch. The call lasted all of about 30 seconds. In that 30 seconds, my entire life flashed before my eyes.

* * *

Up until that moment, I considered myself lucky and fortunate for all that I had received and accomplished in life. I played 16 years in the National Hockey League and made history as the first American-born native son to be drafted by his hometown team in the first round when the Chicago Blackhawks selected me third overall in the 1984 National Hockey League Entry Draft. Ten years later, I was a part of a Stanley Cup championship team with the New York Rangers, ending the franchise's 54-year drought. When it came time to retire in 2000, I had no regrets. Everything I had accomplished professionally came from hockey. It was all I knew.

I was working for NBC as an analyst for NHL games and also doing the same job for the local network televising Blackhawks games.

I also parlayed my passion for betting on thoroughbred racehorses into a TV career with NBC on its coverage of the Triple Crown—the Kentucky Derby, Preakness Stakes, and Belmont Stakes—and other major races. In 2014, Sam Flood, executive producer of NBC Sports and NBCSN, took a chance and hired me as a handicapper because Mike "Doc" Emrick, the network's hockey play-by-play announcer, always asked me for my picks for horse racing events and we would promote it during our hockey coverage. For that, I was eternally grateful. NBC wasn't sure about hiring a "hockey guy" for horse racing and I didn't want to take anyone's gig. I just wanted to add what I could to what they were doing, and it worked out well. I picked some long shot winners in the first two races I broadcast and that really helped boost my profile. NBC was promoting some of my predictions for the Triple Crown races during the hockey broadcasts and people were starting to take notice.

At times, my schedule conflicted with hockey and I had to work an NHL Stanley Cup playoff game and a race, such as the Derby, in the same week. But I couldn't have been happier. Hockey and horses were two things I loved, and I was getting paid to talk about both.

But now I had cancer and had no idea if the chemotherapy would lead to remission. We had no history of cancer in our family and I thought I had been in excellent physical shape. I had taken good care of my body, working out regularly and staying active. I never smoked or drank, which I thought about after that call from Dr. Strong.

You can think you have everything in life, but it doesn't matter if you don't have your health—and at that moment I didn't know what to think.

My world and the world of my family and friends had turned upside down in about seven days.

I had been scheduled to leave from Chicago for New Jersey to work as part of NBC's coverage of the Haskell Invitational—a major thoroughbred horse race after the Triple Crown—on July 30. But a few days before that I started to experience pain on and off in the left side of my abdomen. You get old and your body starts to ache, either because of age or from hockey bumps rising to the surface. But in general I felt good and was in good health, or so I thought.

I woke up and went to the bathroom to take a crap. I was constipated, which was not normal. Diana and the kids were scheduled to visit my father-in-law in Columbus, Indiana, thinking I would be away in New Jersey for the Haskell. I didn't consider my pain serious enough to tell them to cancel their trip.

I wasn't feeling better as the hours went by, so I called my horse racing bosses, producers Rob Hyland and Billy Matthews, to say I didn't feel well and wouldn't be coming to New Jersey. I just had a feeling I should not try to be a hero, even though I felt like I had a great read on the race from a gambling point of view. Laffit Pincay III, my friend and NBC teammate, called and said, "Edzo, you must be really sick to miss this race."

I called my best friend, Dominic Porro, and asked him to buy some Metamucil and come stay with me. If something happened and I needed to go to the hospital, he could take me there and then look after our family's two Labrador retrievers, Lily and Daisy.

The Metamucil didn't relieve the problem and early the next morning I had a fever and started heaving. While still unable to produce a bowel movement, I went back and forth to the bathroom and began vomiting violently. I hadn't used the bathroom for three full days, so I woke up Dominic, who was sleeping in the basement, and told him I needed to go to Lake Forest Hospital.

Once admitted, they detected a blockage in my colon and gave me an enema. They hoped it would clean out my system and that I'd be able to go home in a couple of hours. That sounded good to me because I would be able to bet the horse races on my Xpressbet.com account, which allowed me to wager on races without having to be present at the racetracks.

But the enema barely helped. I was hoping for some major relief, but all I ended up doing was crapping like a rabbit and it was not enough to relieve the pain. The hospital staff did an ultrasound and decided I needed an operation to remove the blockage.

Nobody except Dom knew I was in the hospital because I didn't want to worry anyone. Now I was told I needed surgery. It was like a bad dream. It was about 4:30 AM and I was nervous and scared.

The surgeon came in and told me they wanted to remove a section of my colon and connect it to the outside of my stomach. Immediately I knew it was pretty serious. They wheeled in a video screen to show me male models wearing colostomy bags and told me I'd be wearing one for three months, and then they'd reconnect the colon. I said, "What is going on? Is this really happening? Am I going to have a bag on the side of my stomach for three months?"

Now I was really starting to worry.

Dom leaned over after the doctor left the room and suggested I call the Blackhawks and get some help. I knew immediately I'd contact Dr. Michael Terry, the team's physician. He has helped the Olczyk family with everything from hockey injuries, to our daughter's dancing injuries, to other illnesses. He was always the first person I called when I needed medical help.

I picked up the phone—I guess it was around 5:45 AM local time—hoping he would answer and give me some direction. He was in Michigan, which is an hour ahead, and I apologized for bothering him so early. He asked me what was happening and I told him, so he talked to the attending surgeon and the emergency personnel.

"Edzo," he said, "just tell them you don't want anything done and want to be transported downtown to Northwestern Hospital and I'll start the process."

Once I told the attending personnel I wanted to be sent to Northwestern, they weren't overly pleased. I wasn't their patient anymore and the doctors never returned to my room, so I waited for the ambulance.

I called Nick, who was already awake at the time and fishing, and he awoke Diana. I told her something was really wrong and she said, "We're coming home." She left with Tommy and Nick and it took about four hours to get to the hospital because of traffic. Alexandra was out of town at summer school at the University of Alabama. At that point, we had no idea what would happen next.

DIANA OLCZYK
Eddie's wife

The first thing I thought about when he was in the hospital was, he has a history of kidney stones and blood clots. He was nervous and upset and I knew Dominic had taken him to the hospital, but I was a little perturbed because he hadn't called me until then. I think he'd been in the hospital for hours prior to calling me, but I think he was just waiting for a diagnosis so he wouldn't scare me. He filled me in a little bit that he had blockage, but they didn't know if it was something they could just go in and clean out. Then the doctor came on the phone and scared the living daylights out of me and said he had a tumor and needed surgery. I was just trying to process the information and I said, "Whoa, you're not touching my husband. You need to wait until I get there. We'll be on our way shortly." Eddie came back on the phone and he sounded terrified.

Dr. Terry talked to Dr. Michael Ruchim, a Chicago gastroenterologist who is affiliated with Northwestern. He also called Dr. Strong, chief of gastrointestinal and oncologic surgery and surgical director of the Digestive Health Center, who would be doing the operation, and Dr. Rajesh N. Keswani, a gastroenterologist who is the center's medical director of quality.

DR. MICHAEL TERRY
Blackhawks head team physician

Eddie was scared, no two ways about it. He was there by himself and you could hear it in his voice. He didn't really know what was going on and then someone told him he was going into the operating room. We intervened and changed the game plan a little bit to get him downtown after speaking to Dr. Ruchim. It went from "Everything's fine" to "You need surgery now."

Because it wasn't my arena, my job with Edzo was to get him to the very best people and then to help him translate things and know what to expect. Edzo has been a good friend of mine for a long time and I was just happy to help out.

The drive to Northwestern was really surreal, crazier than anything I'd ever experienced in my life. I'd driven down the Kennedy Expressway a million times as a citizen, hockey player, fan, and TV broadcaster, always upright. Now I was lying down in an ambulance going into the heart of my hometown feeling uncomfortable physically and mentally. I sure got a different view of the city driving in backward.

We arrived at Northwestern and they started the process to see what was wrong with me, beginning with a scan.

By this time, Diana had arrived with Tommy and Nick, and Dr. Strong explained they planned to do emergency surgery to put in a stent to open up a passageway to clean out my system. I drank some prep to make me crap.

Once they put in the stent, I had no control of my bowel for the next 36 hours.

So instead of appearing on TV talking to millions of people about the horse I expected to win the Haskell, I was in a hospital room awaiting surgery.

Dr. Strong told me I had a tumor in my colon but he was not sure it was cancerous. But that's what went through my head. I had no idea about the size of the tumor or how much of my colon needed to be removed. He also said they would try and reconnect the plumbing on the inside to my stomach but there were no guarantees. There was a chance they might have to connect it on the outside, depending on what they found inside. I would have to live with that for a period of time if he could not reconnect the plumbing. Dr. Strong expected the surgery to last more than five hours.

"Just help me, just fix me, do whatever you have to do, and tell me the truth, no b.s.," I said.

That was the last thing I remember saying to him.

I asked Diana if she knew something they might not have told me, but she said she didn't know any more than I did and I believed her. I asked her two or three more times if she was sure. I just knew it was something bad. The team assembled for my surgery. All the medical staff would have filled an NHL dressing room. I met so many people who would be on hand for my surgery. I was lucky and forever grateful for the team that was going to try and help me.

They performed the surgery the next day and it took five-plus hours. They removed 14 inches of my colon and the tumor, which was the size of my fist. As far as I was concerned, it was cancer. It didn't matter if it was the size of a fist or a raisin.

Any surgery is dangerous, but when you're under the knife for that long it's really scary. I can't imagine what my wife or my kids were going through, or my mom and dad, or my brothers, Ricky and Randy. They were all there because that's how close we are. The only person who wasn't there was my mom, and it wasn't because she didn't want to be there. She doesn't move well, and I didn't want her to come. I told her she could come when I was out of recovery.

Once I awoke from the anesthesia, Diana and the kids told me I said some crazy stuff coming out of surgery and to them it was like a comedy show. Meanwhile, my head really ached from the anesthesia.

Dr. Strong told me about the size of the tumor and how much of the colon he removed. They extracted 23 lymph nodes, seven of them tainted. Zero is better than seven, but they said seven is very manageable. Dr. Strong felt the operation went well and all my plumbing was reconnected on the inside. They sent the tumor to the pathologist.

JAY BLUNK
Blackhawks executive vice president
I wanted to personally see Eddie after his surgery. Eddie had always made a point to visit people who were in need. Always selfless and without fanfare, Eddie would quietly slip into a hospital room or place a phone call to someone in desperation. People who needed a lifeline. Those families never will forget his generosity.

When I entered the room that afternoon it was dark with the exception of the Cubs game that flickered on the TV above. We couldn't bring ourselves to discuss the possibility of cancer. We both sat there, trying to stay positive with the great unknown staring us in the face. When I left the room and headed down the hallway, I said a quiet prayer. I was angry and devastated at the same time.

I returned home two days later and felt a sense of relief, even though I didn't know the result of the pathologist's report. Then I received the call from Dr. Strong that would forever change my life and the lives of my wife, my kids, my parents, my siblings, my friends, and my co-workers. This wasn't just about Eddie Olczyk.

* * *

After hanging up the phone, Diana and I began to cry. The kids were downstairs eating dinner and I couldn't give them the news because I wasn't feeling well physically, and mentally I didn't feel strong enough to look them in the eye and tell them what Diana and I had just found out. Diana decided she would tell them.

I came down maybe 20 minutes later and found it hard to talk to the kids even though they already knew what was happening. I felt weak and less of a person, like I'd become a burden and let people down, particularly my family, because they were worried and scared. They were hurting, and there is nothing worse than seeing the people you love hurt because of you. Telling them became the hardest thing, seeing their reaction and knowing I'd affected their lives in a negative way. But how could I control that? I was sick and in shock.

Nick was scheduled to begin his freshman year at Colorado College and didn't want to go, but I told him he had to go. I promised him I would be fine.

I called my folks, my brothers, Dom, and a couple other friends, Joe "The Judge" Casciato and broadcaster Dave Kaplan, and told them what I had been told. I then called John McDonough, the president and chief executive officer of the Blackhawks, and Sam Flood. I also phoned my Blackhawks' TV play-by-play partner Pat Foley and Doc Emrick.

DIANA OLCZYK
Eddie's mother
I was doing a lot of praying. I wasn't angry at God. I believe he had a plan for Eddie and, in fact, I asked God to take away his cancer and give it to me.

ED OLCZYK
Eddie's father
I was in shock. I thought to myself, why not me, why him? He's only in his 50s.

They all knew I had the surgery and that it was serious, but none of them knew what the diagnosis would be. I wanted to make sure they heard the news from me because in the world we live in, news of this kind spreads like wildfire.

That whole night felt like a blur. All of the calls were very hard to make, but everyone I spoke to provided incredible love and support.

By now, people were starting to worry about me because I'd missed the Haskell broadcast and didn't participate in a scheduled charity hockey game and an autograph signing. All I wanted to do was crawl under a rock and not deal with it, but as a public figure I felt I had to do something. We decided to issue a press release through the Blackhawks that would indicate I'd been diagnosed with colon cancer and that I would be undergoing further treatment in the coming weeks, including chemotherapy. The idea was to control the message and let people know I was sick, but that I planned to battle this and worry about everything after that.

"I have been working with outstanding health care professionals and expect to be back in the broadcast booth after I complete my treatment," the release said. "Having the support and encouragement from my family, the Chicago Blackhawks organization, NBC Sports, and all my friends and fans means the world to me and will give me continued strength to beat this. My family and I appreciate privacy during this time as we focus our attention on my treatments."

This was followed by statements from Dr. Terry, John McDonough, and Sam Flood. Collectively, they provided optimism about my return to health and working again. I was grateful for all the well-wishes and support from the hockey and horse racing worlds.

JOHN McDONOUGH
Blackhawks president and CEO

We met the next day after he'd been told. I just wanted to be there for him and let him talk. I told him that I loved him, that the Chicago Blackhawks were completely behind him. Whatever time he needed, it didn't matter. If it was days, months, years, whatever. That support is important when someone receives news like that. You really find out a lot about people, and I think he really needed to know that everybody here was going to be supportive of him. I wanted to have him feel that there was a strong sense of allegiance and comfort.

In an interview with Chris Hine of the *Chicago Tribune*, Doc said, "I read in the *Washington Post* that 75 percent of Americans of all faiths pray at least once a week. So, there is something I/we can do. It makes a difference. I will look forward to our next game [with Edzo] even more than the previous 12 years' worth. I have a great original brother in Indiana, but a second 'brother' in Chicago."

I felt better that we'd gone public, and soon after my phone started blowing up with all these people reaching out to me. I was touched that so many people contacted me in one way or another. I've always tried to make people feel good about themselves, whether it was in the dressing room or the living room. As long as everyone else around me is okay and happy and taken care of, I'm good.

Eddie, who was working as an assistant hockey coach with Bemidji State University, tweeted his thoughts about my situation:

"It has been a very emotional number of days for my family. I'd like to say thanks for the unbelievable amount of support we have received. The hockey world is something we wouldn't trade for anything, and the positivity and encouraging messages that have come our way during this unexpected and difficult time has truly been incredible. My dad is the strongest person I know. He's a fighter to the core and is going to beat this. He's going to go pound for pound with the disease and be standing with his hands in the air at the end as he did (scoring) 361 times in his career. He's said to us for years, 'The true colors of someone, some team, or something are not when times are good, but when times are tough.' He's a phenomenal teacher of the greatest game in the world and will now be showing everyone how he will overcome this obstacle. He'll be back on his feet, in the booth, on the track in no time. This I know."

He received 215 messages, almost 1,600 retweets, and 9,000 likes. Many of the messages offered thoughts and prayers, but one really stood out: "Your dad is one of the main reasons why I watch hockey and became a diehard Blackhawks fan. He's the best commentator in all of sports and I can't imagine watching any of the games this year without the Great Eddie O and Foley having fun calling the game. Your father has had a massive impact on so many people's lives and I pray that your dad has a speedy recovery."

It was an emotionally tough time for Eddie. He and his fiancée, Erika Bozin, had scheduled a party for August 6 to formally announce they planned to get married on August 4, 2018—a year to the day that I was diagnosed with colon cancer. The engagement party, which coincided with Diana's and my 29th wedding anniversary, had already been set and I was in no shape to travel by car because I was beat up from the surgery both physically and emotionally. I stayed at home and everybody else went to the party. I promised them I would be at the wedding in a year's time, even though I didn't know that for sure. I was scared but it was just like, "Okay, I'm going to do everything in my power to be there, regardless if I'm sick or I'm 100 percent healthy."

It would take another four weeks to fully recover from the surgery and meet with Dr. Mulcahy.

I had just kind of been going through life and didn't have a lot of stress aside from the pressure I put on myself to be the best hockey analyst and the best horse racing handicapper I could be. But now I was in for the biggest battle of my life, far more complicated than anything I faced in my hockey career.

But as I had been so many times in my life when facing difficult situations, I was determined to beat the odds.

CHAPTER 2

THE BIRTH OF A RINK RAT

I WAS BORN AUGUST 16, 1966, and named Edward after my father, but I was never called Junior because we have different middle names. He is Edward Zdzislaw and I am Edward Walter, named after my paternal grandfather. I was always Eddie, just like my first son, and when the two of us are together and someone says, "Eddie," we just know to whom they are referring. Early in my pro career I was called Ed, but I always liked being called Eddie. I became Edzo in later years when a teammate of mine in Los Angeles, Kevin Stevens, called me that. I have no idea why, but many people, in particular my broadcasting colleagues in hockey and horse racing, call me that. I'm also called Eddie O.

My last name is pronounced OHL-check, even though some people pronounce it OHL-chuck. I've also heard OHL-cheek, OHL-sezeek, and OHL-sezeeki. My last name has been butchered more times than a brisket at a delicatessen.

I told my daughter-in-law Erika to be prepared for people having a hard time pronouncing her married name. Many people say I need another vowel in my last name.

I am Polish on my father's side. My father was born in Germany after his parents emigrated there from Poland before the start of World War

15

II. After the allies bombed Germany, my father and his parents became displaced persons—called DPs—and had the choice of returning to Poland, which was going to be ruled by Russia, or remain in the West. My grandfather worked a variety of jobs, including in coal mines in Belgium and construction. His wife was Mary, who died at age 24, when my father was four. My father recalls his father telling him she went into the hospital a beautiful woman and was withered away when she died a year or two later. Together they had one other child, also a boy, who passed away. My grandfather remarried a woman named Ana, who had two daughters.

When my father was nine, his parents decided to leave Germany. Their first choice was to move to Australia, because that's where my grandfather's sister and her family lived. The plan changed when the Korean War broke out; Australia was only taking families with a maximum of two children. My grandfather had some friends in Chicago, so they decided to move to America. They lived about a mile away from what is now the United Center, the Blackhawks' home arena.

My mother's name is Diana, the same as my wife—I'll get to that interesting coincidence later on—and she was born and raised in Chicago. She is Italian, and I like to think of myself as being more Italian than Polish. My mother makes great Italian foods such as Pizzelles, which are cookies baked specifically for Christmas; Pistachio cake; meatballs; and lasagna.

My mother was raised by a single mother, Florence, after her husband abandoned them when my mother was only a month old. My mother's grandparents looked after her during the day while their daughter worked. My mother and her parents lived across the street from one another and it was also near where my father lived.

My parents, who are two years apart in age, met at Tuley High School and became high school sweethearts. They married four years later. I was born three years after and grew up in the suburb of Niles. My mother chose my name, which thrilled my father. I also have two brothers: Ricky, who was born four years later, and Randy, born a year after that.

I was called Bozo in a loving way by my parents after the character Bozo the Clown. I was also given the nickname Bigfoot by Ted Nieland, whose son Vince was someone with whom I played hockey. Mr. N came up with the name because I had big feet. I was bigger than most kids my age.

My parents worked super hard doing everything they could for me and my brothers, and all of us played hockey. Ricky graduated from Brown University, where he was captain in his final year, and later graduated from Cornell with a law degree. He worked for the National Hockey League Players Association and later in managerial positions with Edmonton and Carolina. He now works as a pro scout for the Toronto Maple Leafs. Randy stopped playing hockey at about the age of 12, but was active in football and baseball. He is a successful businessman, owning Chicagoland Commercial Real Estate.

My parents installed a lot of discipline, respect, and love in me and my brothers. My dad worked in the grocery business and evolved from a management position into owning his own business, opening his first store on the south side of Chicago when I was 12. Whatever we as kids wanted to do, my parents found a way to support it and make it happen.

My parents both played multiple sports and instilled that passion into us. My father played quarterback in football and was grooming me into becoming the greatest receiver who ever lived. Before dinner, he'd throw me 100 passes in our living room, which was like a playroom because we didn't have any furniture, and if I missed one my dad started all over again. He threw a few that even Mike Ditka would have had a hard time catching. No wonder I didn't play football. My mother was a good softball player. My parents also bowled and golfed.

My journey into hockey began when I was about six and a half. I brought home a pamphlet from school advertising skating lessons. Teachers would regularly send students home with notices about food drives, special lunches, signing up for soccer, and what have you. We must have been sent home with six or seven notices a day from school.

I don't know why I became so interested in learning how to skate; it was just by chance. I asked my mother if I could try skating, but I wanted to get off the ice and quit after my first lesson because my feet hurt. My mother wouldn't let me do it because she paid for the lessons. It was tough love, but had she decided to let me quit, I likely never would have had a career in hockey. My brother Ricky laughs at it now, thinking how my destiny could have changed if our mother allowed me to quit.

Skating turned into learning how to play hockey about six months later. My mother bought me white figure skates, not knowing the difference between figure skates and hockey skates, and in my first practice the coach told her I had the wrong kind. So, my parents bought me new hockey skates for about $25. I received my first set of hockey equipment from the Kelin family, who lived directly across the street from us. They were very heavily involved in the sport with their son, Eddie, and his sister Jill was dating a hockey player on the high school team. The Kelins charged my parents $20 for the equipment and it didn't matter to me that it was used. My parents still have the wooden skate guards and gloves that they bought.

A couple of years later, I went to a bookstore in Niles where Bobby Hull was doing a signing. He was a legend, the Michael Jordan of Chicago in that era. Even though you had Gale Sayers and Dick Butkus of the Bears and Ernie Banks of the Cubs, everyone knew who Bobby Hull was just because of the way he played and his lifestyle. He was always signing autographs. I probably waited in line for four hours to get that autograph. My mother was working at National Tea, a grocery store at the Golf Mill Shopping Center, and the bookstore was around the corner.

Hockey was 24-7 for me. I would get dressed in all my hockey gear and my mother would sing "Here Come the Hawks"—the team's official introductory song—and I'd run around the family room. My mother would play goal wearing a helmet and gloves and my brothers and I would shoot tennis balls at her. I remember doing that hundreds of times and it's a great memory of my childhood, her spending time with me and my brothers and creating and generating the passion of hockey by singing my favorite song.

The Ballard Sports Complex in Niles became a place where I spent a lot of time skating and playing hockey. I'd be a guard for public skating and in the summer, I worked at the batting cage and miniature golf course that would take over the ice.

Nobody ever had to tell me to shoot pucks after school or go to the rink and play shinny or convince my mom to let me play recreational "rat" hockey with the older kids. Once I started playing, I was all-in. I started realizing by my second year of hockey that I was so much better than anyone else.

ED OLCZYK
Eddie's father

People say it is hard to evaluate your kids, but I just tried to put him in where he really fit in. I thought he was head and shoulders above other kids and I just told him that. The parents of the kids he played with in Niles as a young boy were a lot better off than we were. They really didn't want him playing with them. That's why he played with the older kids. He dominated the young guys anyway. That part of his life gave him more drive.

When he started playing with the travel team, the coach didn't know anything about him and had him playing defense. One of the other coaches in the organization said, "What the hell are you doing? Put the kid up front where he belongs." He hesitated a little bit and then progressively moved him up front.

I shot pucks in the basement and garage thousands and thousands of time. I'd shoot until I needed to go somewhere or my hands started bleeding because the stick was digging into the heels of my hands. One day I broke the toe of my stick because it was so worn out and I realized I should be shooting the puck from the middle to the heel of the stick. I started practicing that way and used this practice stick with half a blade. That's one of the reasons I had such a hard, effective shot. Whether it was stickhandling or shooting, I would automatically have confidence every time I had the puck.

Did I think about playing in the NHL when I was eight years old? Probably not. Maybe when I got to 10 or 11, I began dreaming about playing for the Hawks.

My mother remembers a time when I was around that age that we were sitting in the car outside of a McDonald's on Dempster Street in Skokie. It must have been around St. Patrick's Day, because she remembers us having a Shamrock Shake. I had just practiced at Skokie Ice Arena and she told me the coach of our team had been approached by a scout from the Hawks who had been there and asked questions about me. The scout may have been there scouting an older age group, but the coach relayed the information to my mother and she told me about it. My mother said, "Work hard and go for the gold. Just think, Eddie, they're looking out for you."

One time I was asked to try out for the travel team—what some people would call a Triple A team—that was known as the Chicago Jesters. It was intimidating because I was comfortable where I was, but after my first tryout I did so well I realized I could do it and never looked back.

My mother used to get really charged up watching my games, and when someone would say something like, "Get that big kid with the yellow helmet," she took it to heart and said something back. My dad subsequently decided to sit away from her and my mother moved away from the nonsense and name-calling from other parents and stood by the glass.

I was a huge hockey fan—I had posters on the ceiling and the walls of my bedroom, collected hockey cards, pennants, pucks, *GOAL* magazine, autographs, you name it. I lived and died with the Hawks and thought maybe someday I could play for them. Most kids who grow up and cheer for a team, regardless of the sport, always dream about playing for that particular team. Your days are great when they win and aren't so great when they lose. I thought about what it would be like to put that Blackhawks sweater on and realize a dream come true.

My first idol was Bobby Clarke, the captain of the Philadelphia Flyers. I didn't play with anything close to the physicality and grittiness of Bobby, but I had incredible respect for him because of the way he carried himself, his leadership, his faceoff skills, and his competitive drive. He had to overcome the stigma of playing professionally with Type 1 diabetes. That's why he slipped to 17th overall in his draft year despite a great career with the Flin Flon Bombers of the Junior A League in Western Canada.

He was a great faceoff man and I studied him more than any other center. He wore No. 16 and that's the number I had when it was available. In the Olympics, I wore No. 12; my linemate Pat LaFontaine, who was older, wore 16. When I was on the street playing Showdown, the one-on-one skills competition the NHL had, I would imagine being Tony Esposito in goal and Bobby Clarke on the offensive side.

There weren't a lot of kids talking hockey at school. It was more Cubs and Bears. When I'd tell people my age I played hockey, they'd say, "Who does that? Why are you doing that?" It was a much different time then compared to now, much of that due to the 1980 Olympics and how the gold medal won by the U.S. team broadened interest in the sport and spawned youth programs across the country.

I also loved Hawks center Tom Lysiak because of the way he played. He was a great passer, great in the faceoff circle, had a lot of skill, and overall was a super talented guy. He played five and a half seasons with the Atlanta Flames before he was traded to Chicago. I was fortunate to become a teammate of his in the final two years of his career.

When I would go with my dad to the old Chicago Stadium to watch the Hawks play—they weren't broadcast on TV at that time—I'd look at how guys played and try to mimic them or repeat their specific moves or passes. I gravitated toward guys I wanted to play like. I'd see myself in certain aspects of their games, whether it was 10 percent of Bobby Clarke or 55 percent of Tom Lysiak. I just watched their every move.

I also liked watching Hawks center and captain Stan Mikita. He turned his style around 180 degrees, going from a player who fought a lot early in his career to cutting back significantly and winning the Lady Byng Trophy twice for gentlemanly play. Stosh was silky smooth, had great hands and great vision. He wasn't a big guy by any stretch, but he was a tough guy. He was the leader of that team for so long. The numbers and the success that he had were incredible. He could distribute the puck, and his tremendous passing allowed Bobby Hull to become such a great goal-scorer with his slap shot.

I met Stosh for the first time when I was about 14. He had either just finished his Hall of Fame career with the Hawks in 1980 or was hurt. Stan was a man of the people and was just walking around the concourse. The encounter happened in a bathroom at the arena in between periods.

What was he doing there? What does anybody do there?

I was standing right next to him and shook his hand. I ran into him many times since and never thought to mention the first time we met. When I did relate the story about 30 years later, when he and Bobby Hull and Tony Esposito were brought back as ambassadors of the Hawks, he replied, "Did you wash your hands?" That was how quick-witted Stan was. I said to myself, "Yeah, I had hand sanitizer in my pocket 30 years before anybody else did."

We moved as a family to the southwest suburbs of Palos Heights in my early teens because of my father's business. For practices, my mother would drive me to the Oasis Travel Plaza on the 294 tollway, and my father, who was finished working, would take me from there. They'd switch cars and my mother headed home.

The Southwest Ice Arena became my home rink to train and play rat hockey and go for public skating. It was owned and run by Frank DiCristina Sr.—Mr. D—whose son Frankie Jr. was an aspiring hockey player. There was always ice time available when we needed to train or just wanted to play pickup hockey.

I played a lot of golf and baseball as a kid. I loved baseball and still do. I played either pitcher, catcher, or shortstop. When I was 13 years old I played on a traveling team called the Mighty Meteors that played about 100 games a summer. Bob Kabat, whose son, Kurt, I played hockey with, was the team owner. We traveled all around for tournaments, and sometimes we played as many as 12 games on a weekend. That's how intense the schedule could be. He once took us on a friendship tour to Taiwan and the Philippines. That's where I fell in love with shrimp cocktail.

My father believes I could have been a better baseball player than a hockey player. As I know now, dads know best. I do think about it every once in a while, but hockey became a year-round sport and I had to give up baseball when I was 14.

* * *

My interest away from playing sports became thoroughbred horse racing.

It began when I was 12 with Tony Kwilas, who was the manager of our Chicago Minor Hawks team and a horseplayer. His son, Danny, was our goalie. One day I was over at their house in Arlington Heights and they were going to the Arlington Park racetrack, so I joined them.

I became fascinated with the horses, how majestic and pristine they looked on the track, and their competitive nature. Being a person who stood by the rail—someone called a railbird—and watching and learning about the handicapping and the gambling part of it was pretty cool.

The first couple of bets I made using numbers and names, and lost. And then I hit. When I went to cash the ticket, the teller asked me, "How old are you?" I replied, "You didn't ask me how old I was when I lost." The teller looked at me and winked and gave me $118. I gave him a $3 tip.

I don't know why, but I learned quickly. I started watching and learning and asking questions and I went a couple of times in the summer by myself or with some buddies. I can't remember if I was cutting lawns or had an allowance, but I didn't have a lot of money to go to the track.

My father knew what I was doing but my mother didn't, and I'm sure there were a few times I found my way into Mom's purse or Dad's private stash of cash and borrowed a few $20s. If you are going to the track, you'd better have some cake in your pocket.

I remember asking Mr. Kwilas some questions or hearing him talk to one of his buddies about what they liked. Danny had been to the track before with his dad, so he knew a little bit about it.

Years later, I was going to Brother Rice, an all-boys Catholic high school on the south side of Chicago. I had a *Daily Racing Form*, which is the paper that has the entries and results from the races, and at that time was the size of a bedsheet. This was during a time when most kids didn't use backpacks. You just carried your books around and would go to your locker in between classes. I had some classes close together and my locker was at the opposite end of the school, so I carried a bunch of books with me at once.

One time I happened to have the *Daily Racing Form* with me, having handicapped the card the night before. We were in religion class and the brother in the class asked us for our homework. I was going through a folder and the *Daily Racing Form* hit the floor. The next thing you know this big foot lands right on top of it before I could pick it up.

"Olczyk, what's this?" asked the brother, smashing a yardstick on my desk and catching my knuckles. "Are you gambling?"

It was religion class and I couldn't lie.

24

"Not right now," I replied.

Whack with the ruler.

"Do you go to the racetrack?" he asked.

"Every once in a while," I said.

"How do you do?"

We're having this discussion and there are probably 17 or 18 other students in the room.

"Is your *Form* marked up?"

"Yeah, I did my homework," I replied.

"We'll see how good you do. This is my *Form* now," he said.

The *Form* was for that night's card at old Sportsman's Park, and because it was Friday I didn't see the brother again until Monday. The moral of that story is, don't bring your *Daily Racing Form* to religion class or have it marked up. I don't remember how my picks did or whether or not the brother actually bet on them. But he was a tad nicer to me on that Monday. No yardstick in sight.

The *Daily Racing Form* is considered the bible for handicapping the ponies, so when I look back I did bring the bible to religion class, in a way.

CHAPTER 3

THE OLYMPICS

THE WIN BY THE American men's hockey team in the 1980 Olympics left a lasting impression on me. In my opinion it is still the greatest upset in all of team sports. You're sitting there as a 12-year-old kid watching on TV (taped-delayed in some instances), listening live on the radio, or calling a phone number to get the updated info. Being a young hockey player, I thought, how great would it be to play in *that*?

The U.S. winning gold helped put that dream on my radar, perhaps eight or 12 years down the road, but the timetable changed when I received a letter inviting me to the 1984 U.S. Olympic team tryouts taking place at the National Sports Festival in Colorado Springs in July 1983.

But it almost didn't happen because of a series of moves, one in particular that was purely political.

At the age of 14, I attended a local bantam tryout camp that was part of a process taking place throughout the state of Illinois to determine the best players. Those decisions would later factor into which 80 players from various regions across the country would be invited to the U.S. National Player Development Camp in Colorado Springs.

The local tryout camp I went to took place at the Barrington Ice Arena and the organization that was running the camp, the Elmhurst Huskies, was in charge of making all the selections. That organization ran hockey in Illinois. There were about 250 kids at this tryout, and after the first practice, I was cut.

I was devastated, but let's put this in perspective. I was the best 14-year-old hockey player in the United States. Only one player in the world was better at that age—Mario Lemieux—so, yes, the fix was in. I know I was cut because I wasn't affiliated with the Elmhurst Huskies. It was pure politics. But as a 14-year-old, all I knew was that I was cut. I had no idea about politics.

My dad's attitude was that I should play better and there would be better days ahead. Thanks, Dad, good advice. I performed really well at that tryout—there was never a question in my mind that I would make the final camp—but maybe it was a good thing to get my attention.

In 1981, I played in the Midget U.S. Nationals in Tonawanda, New York, and my parents had to borrow $614 from the bank to cover the cost of traveling; my mother still has the promissory note. My brother Ricky was with us and he was cheering for me and my team when he was approached by Len Ceglarski, the legendary coach of Boston College, asking if he was related to anyone playing for the Chicago team. Ricky pointed to me and said I was his brother.

A year later I played in the same tournament and we won it, beating Detroit Compuware. Some people say that Compuware team was the best midget team of all time, featuring future NHLers such as Pat LaFontaine, Al Iafrate, and Alfie Turcotte. But they were not on that day in Manchester, New Hampshire. Our coach, Tim Mueller, gave one of the most moving pregame speeches I ever heard at any level. Even though we had not beaten Compuware all year, he made us believe this was our time to win and pulled out a boom box and played the song "This Is It" by Kenny Loggins. There was not a dry eye in the locker room. There we were, a bunch of 15- and 16-year-old kids, crying in the locker room before the biggest game of our lives.

My parents and I had already decided that I was going to Canada to play my next year of hockey because the competition would be better.

This is something we decided after we had gone to see Bob Pulford, the general manager of the Chicago Blackhawks, to ask his advice about my career. The late Dinny Flanagan, the GM of the Stratford Cullitons of the Western Ontario Jr. B Hockey League, was recruiting me and contacted my parents. Peter Miller, coach of Father Henry Carr of the Metro Toronto Jr. B Hockey League, also wanted me to play for his team.

My folks did some homework, we went on a couple of visits, and I chose Stratford. I was recruited along with two other guys from Chicago, Mark LaVarre and Danny Kwilas.

I decided to make a career decision at 15 because I knew I wanted to play in the National Hockey League. I wasn't sure how to get there, but I knew I was on that path.

* * *

Mark, Danny, and I billeted with a woman for a couple of months until the lady mentioned to Mark that he reminded her of her ex-husband and that we were a little too rowdy for her liking. We packed up and moved and then we split up. Danny and I went to live with Ted and Marion Turford.

Being away from home forces you to grow up pretty quickly. Discipline is needed; I had to get up for school on my own, had my own bank account, and all that kind of stuff. My parents were 890 miles away.

In Stratford, famous as the birthplace of Justin Bieber, everything revolved around hockey. You read about it in the newspaper and saw highlights and reports on TV. It was hockey all the time, so it was right in my wheelhouse. It was a great place to be and great to be a part of a community like that. The arena was a little barn and the crowds were great. I'll be forever grateful to Mr. and Mrs. Flanagan for that opportunity. I was a 16-year-old playing against guys three and four years older, and it was a tough league. Dave Cressman was our coach and overall it was a great experience for a young guy dreaming of playing in the NHL.

We went to the All-Ontario Final against Henry Carr and unfortunately, we lost. I led the team in scoring with 50 goals and 92 assists in 42 games and was voted the league's Most Valuable Player and Rookie of the Year, and was selected the Cullitons' Player of the Year, Most Enthusiastic, Most Impressive Newcomer, and Three-Star Player of the Year.

We had various agents talking to us, but we settled on Bill Watters and Rick Curran, who had a company called Branada Sports Management that represented many high-profile players.

I attended the U.S. National Player Development Camp because Bob Pulford made a call on my behalf to USA Hockey and Lou Vairo, the Olympic team head coach, to make it happen. I made a good impression and subsequently received a letter indicating I had been invited to the Olympic tryouts.

LOU VAIRO
U.S. Olympic team head coach

I get a call from Bob Pulford who said, "This kid can play, he should be at the camp. Trust me." I saw Bob Pulford play a lot and I knew he was a fantastic coach and GM. He didn't have to do any more than say, "Lou, the kid can play, he belongs there." Why wouldn't I take Bob Pulford's opinion?

I'd never heard of Eddie and I'd never seen him play and I still can't pronounce his last name. The first shift, you could see his hockey sense. He was an outstanding player, one of the best I ever had, and I appreciated him. I'd say he was one of the most enjoyable players I'd ever had the chance to see play or to coach. I loved him as a hockey player. I still do to this day. I greatly admire him and am grateful I had a chance to have a front-row seat and watch him.

To me, he was one of the greatest hockey players I ever had the privilege to coach. He was a pleasure to watch as a fan, forget about coaching him. I enjoyed watching him.

It wasn't totally surprising I earned an invitation because of how well I had played in Stratford the year before, and I think Rick Curran and Bill Watters knew that U.S. Hockey was going to grant me an invitation. I wrote on my mattress at home in Chicago that I was going to make the team.

The festival brought together 2,600 athletes from 33 sports for the 10-day event, but the men's hockey team was one of only two sports that would select a team for the Olympics based on what happened in the competition. I remember being really nervous; there were 80 players invited and I was the youngest at age 16. There were some guys who were 10 or more years older than me, and there were some returnees from the 1980 team. Off of the ice I was intimidated because I was around adults. I know some of the players were thinking, what is this high school kid doing here?

The players were divided into four teams and I was on the East squad, coached by Lou Lamoriello, the head coach of Providence College and the school's athletics director, who had selected the younger players. Mr. Lamoriello was great and I'll be forever thankful that I was on his team. Many years later we were inducted into the U.S. Hockey Hall of Fame together. Anytime our paths cross, we still tell the story of that team he put together for the tryout camp. You talk about respecting someone— there are not many people I respect as much as Mr. Lamoriello. He has always had time for me. We always talk family and he always asks how my folks are. He's a first-class human.

The hockey part was the least of my concerns. I had played against some of the other guys such as Pat LaFontaine, Al Iafrate, David A. Jensen, and I knew Chris Chelios because he was from Chicago. I was comfortable in that sense.

It was commonly known that some of the players were going to be selected to the team regardless of what happened in the tryouts. I don't know the exact number, but it was speculated that it was anywhere from 10 to 15 of what would be a roster of 26. I decided I was just going to play my best and hopefully get one of the last remaining spots and see what happened from there.

We practiced and played round-robin games and I finished with four goals and two assists, second-best overall in the tournament. Like I said, I was the most comfortable when I was on the ice.

On July 4, 1983—Independence Day in the U.S. and a day I'll always remember because of how it pertained to my hockey career—all the players were brought into a room and Lou Vairo announced who made the cut. They did it in alphabetical order and eventually they said Edward Olczyk.

You hear your name a thousand times, but to that point I had only been called Edward twice in my life. But when Lou Vairo said it, it was incredible. My heart skipped a couple of beats. It was like, "Holy cow, I did it." Everybody told me I wouldn't make it because I was too young, but I did.

The dorm room floors had one pay phone and I called my mom and my brothers to let them know I made it and they were super excited. My father had attended the tryouts. I called my agents right after that.

Now, it didn't mean I would be playing in the Olympics. That would be determined based on a schedule of 65 games in 44 cities against teams from the National Hockey League, Central Hockey League, American colleges, and national squads from other countries, notably Canada and Russia. Leading up to the Olympics, the roster would be whittled down.

But even making it that far was pretty amazing. What you have to understand is that coming on the heels of the Miracle on Ice and all the notoriety and attention from it, the roster announcement was big news. The 1980 team was comprised of a bunch of college kids and players who weren't known outside of the American hockey community. The victory opened so many doors for U.S. hockey players to play in the National Hockey League—and by this time I knew that's what I wanted to do. If you made this Olympic team, everyone would know your name whether you won the gold medal or not.

But trying to follow what that team did was almost impossible because anything less than that gold medal would be seen as a failure. The expectations were through the roof, but when I was named to the team it was pretty special.

A lot of things went through my mind: back in February 1980 I was dreaming about playing in the Olympics and the NHL. I had left home as a 16-year-old to play in Stratford and then I tried out for the Olympic team and made it. Now I was about to go to Colorado Springs to begin the journey and eventually move to Bloomington, Minnesota, the team's home base, with an eye toward cracking the final roster.

We were given the schedule of where and whom we'd be playing and it began with an early trip to Fairbanks, Alaska. It had an arena similar to the European rinks, which were longer and wider than North American rinks and matched the dimensions we'd be playing on in the Olympics in Sarajevo, Yugoslavia.

We played four games against the Soviet Wings, a touring club team, going 1–1–2. Tom Barrasso, our projected starting goalie, played in the opening game, then received team permission to leave. I think it was for his sister's wedding, and the next thing we know he's in the NHL after signing with the Buffalo Sabres, which had selected him fifth overall in the draft. He went on to win the Vezina Trophy as the NHL's top goaltender and Calder Trophy as Rookie of the Year. Smart move by Tommy B. Our goalies became Marc Behrend and Bob Mason.

Fairly early into the process, I was placed on a line with center Pat LaFontaine, who was excused from the tryout because he was exhausted from playing in his first season in Major Junior A, and left wing David A. Jensen. We were dubbed the Diaper Line—I think defenseman Chris Chelios, who wasn't much older, came up with it—because we were so young. We had immediate success in the series against the Soviet Wings, scoring a bunch of goals.

Then we played some games in Finland before finally moving to Bloomington. I'd just turned 17 and now I was playing against professionals and minor-pro guys, the latter having the same hopes and dreams that we all did of playing in the NHL. Those games helped prepare me and a lot of guys for the next level. You're playing against men and seasoned pros. The Central Hockey League schedule was pretty tough and it counted in the standings.

Wherever we went it was a circus—lunches with mayors, keys to the city, and all kinds of appearances—because of the connection to the 1980 team. When we went into a town, it was hyped up that the U.S. men's Olympic hockey team was coming, and we'd stop traffic. We got a lot of attention and a lot of fanfare that went with it. Looking back, someone should have had the understanding it was too much on certain occasions. They should have picked better spots because they ran us ragged off the ice.

We traveled to the White House, where we met President Ronald Reagan. I have a couple of photos on my mantel at home of me standing next to the president in the Rose Garden. It was surreal—a 17-year-old kid shaking hands with the president of the United States—and he's shooting a puck into a net against Marc Behrend. It was an incredible honor to have that opportunity and celebrate USA Hockey, all thanks to the 1980 team. Anytime you get an opportunity to get honored at the White House with a standing president, that's a huge honor and privilege.

We played a series against the Russians in December in Lake Placid and the town was awash in memories of the Miracle on Ice. In his autobiography *Made in America*, Chris Chelios wrote, "The entire town of Lake Placid was fired up for the game. People in cars were honking their horns. Everyone had their flags out. People wanted to relive the 1980 moment. It seemed more like a Stanley Cup Final game than an exhibition game. It was a storybook kind of night."

We were leading 4–2 in the third period after Chelios scored with 5:09 to go. Then the Russians mounted an attack, scoring 48 seconds later and adding another with 1:49 remaining. We won on a goal 31 seconds later by Phil Verchota, who had scored earlier in the game, with his second on a 60-foot pass from Chelios.

"Bedlam ensued," Chelios wrote in his book. "Fans reacted as if we had captured an Olympic medal and we hadn't won anything. These were good players, but none of them would be on the Olympic team. We had beaten the Soviet JV team. Still, it was the most exciting win over a JV squad I'd ever experienced."

In the six-game series, we went 3–2–1. It was big news in the media, including national publications. It is Lou Vairo's opinion that we may have peaked in that series. Overall, we had a record of 39–18–8 in the 65-game schedule. I totaled 21 goals and 47 assists in 62 games.

In our final tune-up against Canada in Milwaukee, Wisconsin, we pounded them 8–2. Looking back that may have been the worst thing that ever happened, knowing they were our greatest competition and we had them in the opening game for both teams in the Olympics.

*　*　*

It was eye-opening to be at the Olympics. Here I was, trying to become a member of a group of players hoping to duplicate what the 1980 team did. Once I set foot in Sarajevo, it was like, "Here we are, this is it. You are in the Olympic Village."

In the brackets determining the two divisions for the 12 nations competing in the tournament, we were included with Canada, Czechoslovakia, Finland, Austria, and Norway. We knew that to have any chance of advancing to the medal round we'd have to beat Canada.

We played our first game the day before the opening ceremonies. We were assembled to be ready more than three hours before the 1:30 PM start. As soon as we boarded the bus, everything went wrong. The driver got lost en route to the arena and then got caught behind the Olympic torch bearer. We arrived about 30 minutes before the opening faceoff. It was a complete gong show. In addition to being late, Pat LaFontaine was running a temperature and some of the guys were suffering from food poisoning from the sausages and burgers the night before. It just could not have been any worse. No excuses, just the facts.

You can argue all you want about the Russians, but I've always believed that Canada has always been our archrival in hockey, and here we were playing them in the first game and everything had started off wrong.

The Canadians scored at 27 seconds of the opening period on a tip-in by Pat Flatley. We tied it up about 10 minutes later on a goal by David A. Jensen. Canada scored on a power-play goal by Carey Wilson about two minutes later. Wilson scored his second goal of the game early in the second to go up 3–1. David scored again, a power-play goal on which Chelios and I drew assists. But Wilson completed a hat trick in the third and the game ended 4–2.

It was almost like we got there, the game was over, and we blew it. You train and sacrifice all that time and pound Canada into submission in the last game we played against them, and then they turn the tables and we couldn't respond.

In his book, Chelios wrote, "Did the pressure get to us? Were we too nervous? Who knows? But we didn't have it that day and we let the loss overwhelm us."

Canada did something different than it had in previous games by employing Dave Tippett to shadow Pat. Obviously Tip was a very good defensive specialist in his career. Canadian coach Dave King made a difference in that game. Losing to Canada was a sign of things to come. It was just a huge letdown.

The next day the opening ceremonies took place in Kosevo Stadium, and it included 1,200 athletes from a record 49 countries competing in 39 events. I can't speak for anybody else on the U.S. hockey team, but the opening ceremonies were very much tainted because of the loss the day before. That said, it was an incredible experience because the whole world is watching and you are walking in with the greatest amateur American athletes.

We were dressed in Western garb that included a cowboy hat, a big belt buckle, and jeans provided by Levi's, the official clothing sponsor of the United States in the Olympics. We were led in by the Norwood Fire

Dept. Band from Lake Placid playing "When the Saints Go Marching In" and carrying the Olympic flag from 1980. It was a great experience to walk in with my hockey teammates and the other American athletes. Overall, it seemed like a long procedure from leaving the Olympic Village, getting to the stadium, taking part in the ceremonies, and then going back. I'd say it was probably a five-hour ordeal. It's tiring physically, but when you are in the moment and knowing this may be your only chance to complete in the Olympics with the world's greatest athletes, it's special.

We played our second game against Czechoslovakia, which beat Norway 10–4 in its opener. After the Canada loss, this was a must-win for us if we hoped to make it into the medal round. The Czechs opened the scoring at 12:23 of the first period with a shorthanded goal. The lights went out in the arena shortly thereafter, causing a half-hour delay. We tied it up two minutes after play resumed on a goal by Mark Kumpel. Overall, the game turned into a penalty-filled contest for both teams—we had 10 minors and the Czechs seven—and they cashed in on two power-play goals. They added another goal in the third period and won 4–1. All I remember is we lost our discipline and took some bad penalties.

We had been pretty disciplined as a team for the most part, but we lost our composure at that point, spending too much time in the penalty box. I don't care what era or tournament you're in, you're chasing the game when you take penalties.

The crowd started to taunt us with anti-American chants. Considering we were the defending champions, everybody was against us. Who in the world isn't against Americans? When something bad happens, we're always the first ones to come to people's aid and also the first to be public enemy number one. That's just life, but when we were there, we knew the crowds weren't exactly pulling for us.

Once you do the math and understand what needs to take place, you realize the chances of getting into the medal round have gone by and you've pretty much got no chance. I was a young kid and I felt that, but we still had games to play. It's just unfortunate the perfect storm went the wrong way.

We played Norway to a 3–3 draw in our third game, in which I scored a power-play goal. We crushed Austria 7–3 after that, and our line had a good game. Pat had a hat trick, David had two goals and an assist, and I had four assists. We tied Finland 3–3 and finished off beating Poland 7–4, in which I scored my second goal of the tournament. We finished seventh overall.

We were prepared and had a perfect schedule. We had everything we needed. You can always look back and wonder how the wheels fall off. Were we able to make adjustments? I can't remember, but when you lose and you are expected to have success, the scrutiny will be there. People have said the team was too young, the coach was inexperienced, there was no discipline, and the best goalie left early in the training camp process. That kind of second-guessing comes with the territory. Unfortunately for us, our best players at the Olympics were our youngest players. That ended up being one of the downfalls. Everything started with that first game—that set the tone—and we obviously didn't have the nuts to overcome that loss. There was plenty of blame to go around. It's easy to blame Lou and the staff, but at the end of the day it comes down to the guys going out there and figuring it out.

When we returned to Minnesota, there was basically nobody there to greet us, the complete opposite of the big sendoff we got when we left. We felt like we let everybody down. We just did not play our best hockey at the most crucial point of the year—and that was the most disappointing part. You leave and the expectations are through the roof—everybody wanted to be a part of the team—but you come home and say, "Holy jeez, we're an afterthought."

We came up short, but life goes on and you live to fight another day. My focus would now be on life after the Olympics.

CHAPTER 4

COMING HOME

IMMEDIATELY AFTER THE OLYMPICS, I had the option of playing for the Toronto Marlies of the Ontario Hockey League, the Laval Voisins of the Quebec Major Hockey League, or the Portland Winter Hawks of the Western Hockey League, all of whom had drafted me and owned my rights.

Playing for Laval would have made me a teammate of Mario Lemieux, the player assumed to be chosen first overall in the 1984 NHL draft. Some of my Olympic teammates joined NHL teams that had drafted them. Only defenseman Al Iafrate and I were eligible for the 1984 NHL draft, and Al chose to join the Belleville Bulls of the OHL. I decided to stop playing instead of going to play more hockey after the Olympics; I figured playing could only hurt my draft status and I also didn't want to risk getting injured. My agents, Bill Watters and Rick Curran, believed that and I respected their advice. Ultimately it was my decision and my parents agreed and supported me.

The Blackhawks brought me in for a home game to drop the puck for the ceremonial faceoff. Philadelphia Flyers captain Bobby Clarke, my boyhood idol, and Hawks captain Darryl Sutter were the two players involved. It was Clarke's final year of his Hall of Fame career. Not sure about the sport coat I had on when dropping the ceremonial faceoff. Maybe I had it on inside out.

On June 7, 1984, my parents flew with me to Montreal before the biggest day of my life, for the draft to be held two days later at the Forum, one of the shrines of hockey.

When we arrived, we traveled around town and had a nice dinner that night. I could hardly wait for the draft because it was something I had dreamed of all my life. Now it was about to become a reality.

One of the coolest experiences happened after going to dinner with my family. I went by myself to visit Bill Watters and Ricky Curran to get the latest rumors and lowdown on the draft. When I arrived back at the hotel, the Manoir le Moine just down the street from the Forum, I was going to the elevator and here comes baseball great Pete Rose, Charlie Hustle, a legend on and off the field.

I had heard the rumors of his liking to get his feet wet with a wager or 10. He was a noted big-time horseplayer. A pro athlete who loved the track is my kind of guy. On this occasion, he was not alone. In horse racing terms, he had a filly on each arm. After a 2–1 win by his Montreal Expos over my Chicago Cubs, Charlie Hustle did not play in the game but he went 2-for-2 postgame. I held the door for the trio and said, "Hey, Mr. Rose." He responded, "Hey, kid, thanks." The elevator came and it wasn't exactly very large, so I passed on trying to squeeze my way in with the trio. I was told he was living at the hotel, or so the legend goes.

The next day my family and I talked to Ricky and Bill and had an idea that New Jersey, picking second overall, was interested in drafting me because I had gone to New Jersey on a visit about six weeks prior to the draft. I met with general manager Max McNab, owner Dr. John McMullen, and was ushered around by legendary NHL executive Marshall Johnston, who was the team's assistant GM. He actually took me to a Mets game as well during my visit. To this day, Mr. Johnston is a great guy. Knowing I am a huge Cubs fan, he would bust my chops for years after about them not being able to win the World Series. Proudly, he has stopped now that there's no more ammo.

Chicago was picking sixth, but Ricky and Billy said there was no way I was going to fall that far. They said the only way the Hawks could get me was to move up. We knew L.A., which was picking third, wanted a defenseman. We weren't sure about Toronto, which was picking fourth.

Yeah, I thought about playing in my hometown, but whatever happened was okay. I just wanted to play in the NHL, the best league in the world.

The Penguins selected Mario as expected, and even though it was anticlimactic it was still a big deal because he was French Canadian and the draft took place in his home province. Mario was expected to be a generational player, following along the lines of Wayne Gretzky in terms of future greatness.

New Jersey selected forward Kirk Muller of the Guelph Platers, and I was disappointed because I thought I'd be second overall.

The time after the Devils' pick seemed like forever. There was a timeout on the floor and Bill leaned over to me and said, "Something's happening." But we had no idea what.

And then it was announced by NHL commissioner John Ziegler that a trade had been made and Chicago had moved up to the third pick overall. Hawks general manager Bob Pulford sent goalie Bob Janecyk, a Chicago guy, and a third-round pick to Los Angeles; the two teams also swapped first-round picks. The Hawks also sent forward Rich Preston and defenseman Don Dietrich to the Devils and acquired forward Bob MacMillan. That trade was made for the Devils not to draft me second overall, whether they wanted me or not. That's the business.

The next thing you know, Hawks assistant general manager Jack Davison grabbed the microphone and announced my name.

I was staying home. My hometown team drafted me. I was a Hawk.

I thought about all those games I went to at the Chicago Stadium as a kid with my dad. I thought about my friends, my family, all those hours at rat hockey, and all the people who helped me, teammates and coaches.

All those hours, thousands of them, shooting pucks in the garage and basement.

It was just a blur.

I remember hugging my mom and my dad and Ricky and Bill. Al Iafrate, my Olympic teammate, was sitting there in the same row because he was also represented by Bill and Rick and was waiting to be drafted (he would go fourth overall). I was in such shock going down from the stands to the floor and over to the Hawks' table because I really did not have any inkling it would happen. I dreamed of playing in the NHL; now I'd be playing for my hometown team.

The Hawks had never selected a hometown player that high in the draft, so I became a part of history. In addition, no American team in NHL history had selected a hometown product in the first round of the NHL draft, so it was another landmark moment. I am so proud of that.

We did a conference call with the media and I was asked what it was like to be drafted by my hometown team. Growing up in Chicago and living and dying with the Blackhawks, I couldn't believe I would now be playing for them and wearing their sweater. All those years sitting in the stands at the Chicago Stadium, looking through the glass at the ice, hearing that famed organ, the horn that blared after a Hawks goal, and Wayne Messmer singing the national anthem, and now I was going to be playing there and walking up those old steps from the dressing room to the ice level.

We tried to fly home the next day but were delayed about 10 hours because of a mechanical issue with the plane and didn't arrive home until 8:00 PM Chicago time. It didn't matter, I was living a dream—or at least starting another. I didn't know when the contract would be done, but I had no worries because Bill and Ricky told me it was going to happen.

RICK CURRAN
Eddie's agent

I think Bob Pulford felt having a kid like that out of Chicago would be great. I'm sure that's why he moved in that direction. To give Eddie credit, he was as mature as any 18-year-old client I had ever had. He'd been through the Olympics and all the fuss and fanfare of the Diaper Line. It wasn't that Eddie wasn't used to that kind of pressure or attention.

BOB PULFORD
Blackhawks general manager

We felt it was very important for our team to get Eddie. We thought he had a chance to be a superstar in the league and him being from Chicago, we felt if we didn't get him we would get criticized for it.

We had made a deal with Los Angeles substantially earlier to move up in the draft to third overall. We had the third choice and thought no one knew it, but New Jersey, which had the second overall choice, found out we had the third pick and they put two and two together. They told us if we made a deal they wouldn't touch Eddie Olczyk with their choice. They kind of blackmailed us. I told Jack Davison, if we don't get Olczyk and he becomes a star, we'll get really crucified.

He had shown he was a good hockey player. We felt we were safe at three in the draft and probably would have been if New Jersey hadn't found out about it. I don't think they were going to take Olczyk anyway, but they were able to scare us enough that we made a deal so they wouldn't take him.

The Canada Cup, an international tournament involving players representing Canada, the U.S., Sweden, the Soviet Union, Czechoslovakia, and West Germany, was taking place in the fall in various Canadian cities and Buffalo. I had a pretty good idea I was going to be invited to the Americans' training camp. So, before I would actually begin my pro career, I was going to have a taste of what it was like to represent my country again only six months after the Olympics, but this time against the best of the best at the pro level.

I was at Team USA's training camp in Montreal when Rick and Bill finalized the contract with Chicago and I flew home the next day for the press conference. I received a Hawks jersey and a hat, and when I shook hands with Pully, who had played a huge role in my career and my life, it really clicked in I would be playing for my hometown team. I would be given No. 16, which had been worn by Rich Preston. Hawks great Bobby Hull wore No. 16 early in his career before switching to No. 9.

The Hawks gave me a four-year deal that paid me $75,000 the first year, $85,000 the second, $95,000 the third, and $105,000 the final year. I also received a signing bonus of $25,000.

At the press conference, Pully talked about how it was a proud day for the Hawks and amateur hockey in Chicago.

"Ed is with the U.S. team preparing for the Canada Cup," he told the media. "I watched him the other night and it made me pretty proud to know we have him on our team. I talked after the game to Lou Vairo, his coach with the American Olympic team and the assistant coach for the U.S. Canada Cup team. In Lou's estimation, Ed will be a 50-goal scorer in the National Hockey League in a few years and for many years after that. He's also a great playmaker and he's physical. The only thing he has to improve is his skating, but he gets there."

I had a prepared speech I had written after I had come home from Montreal. I talked about how this was a day of excitement, joy, and happiness. While I was extremely emotional and cried, I also jokingly referred to North Carolina star Michael Jordan, who had been drafted by the Chicago Bulls, also third overall. This was the first and only time Eddie Olczyk and Michael Jordan were mentioned in the same sentence.

"It's nowhere near the kind of money Michael Jordan will be making when he signs with the Bulls, but this is the biggest moment of my life, even bigger than making the Olympic team," I said. "I want to say thank you to all my teammates from the time I learned to skate all the way up to the U.S. Olympic team, the opposing players I've come in contact with, the coaches and managers I've played for. These are the people who have taught me the skills I needed to have a hockey career."

It was at this point that I became emotional as I began to talk about my family.

"Most importantly, I want to thank my dad and my mom and my brothers, Ricky and Randy, for being there day or night and good and bad. I've been away from you these past two years. But I plan on being here with you for many years to come as a member of the Chicago Blackhawks.

"All the people I've mentioned have touched my life in their own special way, and I hope to give back to them that same special feeling. This is just the first step. The next is making the team.

"It doesn't matter where I play, I feel I can put the puck in the net and I'm very good on faceoffs. I've always had double the number of assists as goals. I'd rather get an assist than score a goal any day.

"I realize I have to earn the fans' respect. Ever since I was a little kid, I dreamed about coming up those flights of stairs in the Chicago Stadium and hearing the greatest fans in the world. I was almost an oddball in school. Nobody played hockey. To be somebody, you had to play football and basketball, but I just loved to play hockey and I always wanted to be a Blackhawk."

Life was pretty good, to say the least.

Team Canada's roster included many of the Edmonton Oilers who had just won the Stanley Cup. My teammates on the final roster were Bob Brooke, Aaron Broten, Neal Broten, Bobby Carpenter, Chris

Chelios, Dave Christian, Bryan Erickson, Mark Fusco, Tom Hirsch, Phil Housley, David A. Jensen, Mark Johnson, Rod Langway, Brian Lawton, Brian Mullen, Joe Mullen, Mike Ramsey, Gordie Roberts, Bryan Trottier, Tom Barrasso, and Glenn "Chico" Resch. I felt fairly lucky to have made the squad because there were some talented players who were cut or couldn't play because of injuries, including Pat LaFontaine. I was the youngest player on the team. Badger Bob Johnson, head coach of the Calgary Flames, was our head coach.

We had a wide range of older, seasoned veterans on our team. There were guys I watched on TV or read about, and all of a sudden I was playing with them. I was intimidated, for sure, but that's just natural. I was going up against the best players in the world.

The format was a round-robin in which each team played five games and the top four advanced to the playoffs.

The Soviet Union finished first overall with a 5–0 record. We placed second with a 3–1–1 record, followed by Sweden (3–2), Canada (2–2–1), Czechoslovakia (0–4–1), and West Germany (0–4–1). We played Sweden in Edmonton in one of the semifinals and lost 9–2. Canada defeated the Soviet Union 3–2 in the other semifinal in Calgary. Canada went on to win the series, winning the best-of-three in two games.

Now it was time to go back home and begin skating with my teammates and wearing the Hawks jersey.

CHAPTER 5

EDDIE OLCZYK, CHICAGO BLACKHAWK

I HAD A LOT OF CONFIDENCE going into that first training camp with the Hawks. There was a lot of attention on me from the media and I definitely felt the pressure. I was both nervous and excited. The Hawks were coming off a disappointing season, so I had to grow up pretty quickly. It was like, "I'm playing for my hometown team and I can't screw this up."

I was mentally tough at that point, but this was no dream. There were guys trying to kick my ass and take my job or keep their job. That's when you realize this is a business. Everybody is friendly and most hockey guys are the greatest guys in the world, but when some 18-year-old punk from Chicago is coming in trying to take your job, that's a different story.

From day one I always felt like I had 36,000 eyeballs on me every night because I was a Chicago guy. I wanted to do so well for so many people, which was no easy task.

After our first preseason game, our head coach, Orval Tessier, told the media I was going to be a great player, referencing my play in the Olympics and Canada Cup. "If he can play that well against the best in the world, he can play for the Chicago Blackhawks," he said.

I learned very quickly that the trainers on a hockey team are the lifeline of a player. They are overworked and underpaid, but they are the best. If you are good to those guys, you are golden forever. I loved those guys my whole career, every one of them.

I had told Hawks medical trainer Skip Thayer during training camp about this dream I had when I was younger. In the dream, I was late arriving to the arena for the first game and security at the players' entrance wouldn't let me in because they didn't know who I was. I would eventually wake up in a cold sweat. I had this dream hundreds of times.

On my way to the arena for the actual game, there was a traffic jam. I was driving my father's car, which had broken windshield wipers. When I arrived at the Stadium, the person at the security entrance prevented me from going in to park. When I told him I was Eddie Olczyk, he said Eddie Olczyk had already arrived.

I couldn't believe what I'd just heard.

I told him I had already played four preseason games and that I was late for my first game in the show. I was beginning to panic and I told the security person to call the Hawks dressing room. Eventually, they let me in. My nightmare had actually come true. I was thinking I was a psychic.

As I was walking, stunned, by the training room, I saw Skip and he said, "Hey, kid, did you have any trouble getting in?"

At that point, I knew Skip had pranked me. Nothing is sacred in a locker room.

I began the season playing right wing on a line with center Tommy Lysiak and left wing Darryl Sutter. I told Tommy that I wrote a letter to him when I was 15 telling him I was a fan of his and that I wanted to play in the NHL. He sent me back a photo of himself that he signed, "To Eddie O, maybe we could play together, Tommy Lysiak." Sure enough, three years later, I was playing on a line with him in my first game. What are the chances of that? To me, that's an incredible story.

When I told him the story, in typical Tommy fashion, he said, "How many other players did you send letters to?" Sadly, Tommy passed away on May 30, 2016. It happened during the Stanley Cup Final between Pittsburgh and San Jose. I travelled to Georgia to pay my respects to his wife, Melinda, and their entire family.

That first game, which was against Detroit, felt different than anything I had experienced to that point. It was a game I had dreamed about my whole life and then all of a sudden here I was, putting on that sweater with my name on the back and walking up those stairs to the ice level and the crowd is going crazy. It was like, man, you've arrived. I thought about my folks, who were there at the game along with my brothers. You have all these people watching you.

Being on the ice and seeing the crowd through the glass was totally different compared to how I had seen the game as a spectator. It was surreal. We won 7–3 and I scored. Every young hockey player dreams of scoring their first NHL goal so they can keep the puck and talk about it after their career and provide the details. Here's how mine happened: Troy Murray passed the pack to Dave Feamster, who shot it from the point. I was cruising in front of the net and the puck hit the end boards and came back out. Red Wings goalie Greg Stefan turned and was out of his net and I put it home while I was getting knocked down on my ass.

The crowd went nuts chanting my name, "Edd-ie, Edd-ie." I could never have imagined that would happen. It was pretty special. I remember they used to do that for goalie Tony Esposito—"To-ny, To-ny"—when he made a great save. I remember thinking I must have done something right for the fans to chant my name.

Keith Brown grabbed the puck and gave it to me and I skated off the ice. I remember raising my right arm and pumping my fist in the air. I couldn't believe it: I had scored a goal in my first NHL game.

RICKY OLCZYK
Eddie's brother

To see him standing on the ice in a Blackhawks sweater for his first game, I kept pinching myself and saying, "This is unbelievable. How blessed are we to see our brother playing?" It was a special night, for sure. To see him score, it was almost like a storybook ending.

After the game I was pulled in every direction by the media. The late broadcaster Tim Weigel, who was a legend in Chicago, did an interview with me from the bottom of the stairs. I had a shiner and stitches in my cheek from the preseason and I couldn't believe this was all happening.

Every game I played, whether it was good or bad, there was hometown pressure. It's just the way it was. There was no doubt some of my teammates, particularly the older guys, were not happy with the attention I was receiving, but it wasn't like I asked for it. This was a story that had never happened before. Think of a kid from Toronto playing for the Maple Leafs, that kind of stuff is pretty normal. Same thing with a kid from Massachusetts playing for the Bruins. This had never happened before in the first round with the Hawks. I wasn't the first native of Chicago to play for the Hawks, but I was the first one selected so high in the draft. I'll always be proud to say where I'm from and this was just something that became part of my NHL learning curve. I definitely had to earn the respect in the locker room.

I always tried to answer my fan mail, something I still do today. When I was with the Olympic team, I received a letter from Kenny Albert, whose father, Marv, is a broadcast legend, and I sent him back an autographed photo. Who knew years later we'd both be working for NBC on hockey broadcasts?

Orval moved me from Tommy Lysiak's line to a line with Curt Fraser on left wing and Troy Murray at center. We meshed right away because we thought the same way and had great chemistry off the ice. Troy is still one of my best friends. We had everything on our line: toughness in Fras, Troy's two-way play, and I was kind of the playmaker and offensive guy.

TROY MURRAY
Eddie's teammate

There was a lot of media attention that normally wouldn't be there for a first-year NHL player because he was playing in his hometown. It was tough, but I thought he handled it extremely well. I don't think the guys on the team were jealous or intimidated by the attention he received, but I think it was a good opportunity to give him a hard time in a nice way. The NHL was always kind of a playful league at that time. Eddie was a very confident young man, and the way that he carried himself was important. He didn't demand people look at him or notice him.

Hawks TV play-by-play man Pat Foley dubbed us the Clydesdales Line because we each weighed more than 200 pounds and there were very few lines at that time that had three guys that big. He just thought it was descriptive for that time, which was when Budweiser had a national advertising campaign featuring Clydesdale horses. Pat says he was trying to be minimally creative, but it became quite popular. The first time I became aware of it was from my parents. Just for the record, we were the fastest Clydesdales around. I think it's still one of the top 10 greatest names for a hockey line.

Back in the day when guys played together for long stretches of time, they were given names: the Production Line, the Punch Line, the GAG Line, the Triple Crown Line, the Trio Grande Line, and the French

Connection, for example. Chicago always seemed to have lines with great nicknames: the MPH Line (Pit Martin, Jim Pappin, and Bobby Hull), the Scooter Line (Doug Mohns, Stan Mikita, and Ken Wharram), the Pony Line (Max Bentley, Doug Bentley, and Bill Mosienko), and the Million Dollar Line (Hull, Murray Balfour, and Bill Hay).

Sometimes during a stoppage in play when I came on to the ice with Troy and Fras, the Stadium organist, Nancy Faust, would play "My Hometown" by Bruce Springsteen. My brother Ricky recalls it being intentional and how he picked up on it right away.

Early in February, with the team sitting in second place in the Norris Division with a record of 22–28–3, Pully fired Orval and took his place as our head coach. Two seasons before, the Hawks finished first in the Norris Division with a record of 47–23–10, second overall in the Clarence Campbell Conference behind Edmonton. The Hawks were swept by the Oilers in the conference finals. Edmonton won the first two games by a combined score of 16–6 and when asked about it after the second game, Orval said, "We'll probably call the Mayo Clinic for heart transplants."

The previous season, the Hawks plummeted to fourth in the division with a record of 30–42–8 and lost to Minnesota in the division semifinals. Looking back, when we started off the season slowly, it was only a matter of time before Orval was fired.

When it happened, I was like, "Okay, the coach gets fired, just keep playing." Pully was a tough guy but the best coach I ever had. He knew what guys could do and couldn't do—old-school strategy!

* * *

Things were going well for me professionally, and personally my life was about to change.

Following an afternoon game at home against Minnesota, we were scheduled to fly to New York for a game the next day against the Rangers. After the game, on the Kennedy Expressway between the old Chicago

Stadium and O'Hare International Airport, there was a brutal accident. The highway was pretty much shut down. We were scheduled to fly via commercial flight on American Airlines and they were not about to hold it back for any late passengers. I was freaking out because I'm a rookie and you don't want to miss a flight. That's the last thing you want to do. I probably committed about 30 vehicle infractions on the way to the airport. I got there, but half the team missed the flight.

We boarded the plane, maybe a dozen players and some staff, and there was this stunning flight attendant taking the boarding passes. I looked at her name tag and it said Diana. I was thinking, wow, that's my mom's name. It was a big plane that was nearly empty and I kind of scoped out the section where she was working and went over to that area by myself. I was thinking, okay, how do I map this out? It's a two-hour flight to New York. How can I get to know her on this plane?

We had a little small talk and I ordered about eight orange juices so she would keep coming back to my seat. She told me her last name was Vickers and I'm thinking to myself, Vickers? The street I live on is McVickers. I'm an Eddie, she's a Diana. My dad's an Ed, my mom's a Diana. This is kind of crazy.

I subsequently found out she had been called by the airlines that Sunday morning to fly from New York to Chicago. She didn't work the flight, she dead-headed, which is the terminology used by the airlines for crew members, pilots, or cabin crew who aren't scheduled to work. She had about 45 minutes to get to the airport. She could have easily missed that flight or not gotten the call, or I could have been stuck in traffic and never made that flight.

I think it was meant to be. Diana said there was an instant physical attraction. Agreed. Call it love at first flight.

We talked and I asked her if she wanted to go to the Rangers game the next day. She said yes and I got her two tickets and told her she could pick them up at the box office. I told her I would meet her there after the game and we exchanged phone numbers. We won 4–3—Behn Wilson

53

scored in overtime—and I showered and walked upstairs in about 10 minutes and went over to the box office area but didn't see her. I walked around Madison Square Garden twice in the pouring rain just to see if I could find her. I had no idea if she picked up the tickets.

She lived in New York and I didn't want to call her apartment that night, so I called the next morning and a guy answered the phone. Yes, a guy; my mind was going a mile a minute. I asked if Diana was there and I was told she was out of town. I asked if she had gone to the hockey game last night and the guy said he wasn't sure. I told him to tell her Eddie called.

I left some messages but there was no communication for a couple of days. She had left me a message on my phone line but I hadn't told her I still lived at home because I didn't want to kill the vibe, something she still laughs about today. My mom asked me, "Who keeps calling at 2:00 in the morning?" I was 18 years old and didn't know how old Diana was. I knew she was a little older, but didn't realize she was 23 turning 24.

Diana had played field hockey at Hanover College, where she was a theatre major, and her brothers, Mike and Tim, had played ice hockey recreationally growing up. She knew the game, but I always tease her by saying the reason she never called me was because she wanted to know if I was indeed a professional hockey player. I joke that she was trying to look up my profile in the days before the Internet. She said she bought *The Hockey News* every week after we met.

When Diana and I finally talked again, she told me she hadn't gone to the game. The airline had put her on reserve because she didn't have much seniority, so she had an opportunity to go home and visit her folks in Columbus, Indiana. I'm thinking, that's real nice. You give me the nine of hearts. It cost me $135 for the tickets.

We played in Vancouver six days later in the first of a three-game road trip. The light on the phone in my hotel room was blinking. It was a message from Diana. I couldn't believe it. I started searching frantically for a pen and paper to write down her number but couldn't find either one. I went to the bathroom and grabbed a bar of soap and wrote her phone number on the mirror. I can't remember if my roommate was there or not. I knew it was late back east and I didn't want to be rude, so I didn't call. Remember, there were no cell phones in 1985. I couldn't sleep a lick and called in the morning and a woman answered saying Diana had just gone out on a five-day trip somewhere in Aruba or Cancun.

Diana and I finally had our first date the day before my first playoff game at Barnaby's Pizza in Des Plaines and hit it off.

I finished the regular season with 20 goals and 30 assists in 70 games, missing 10 starting in late December when I suffered a broken foot taking a Doug Wilson slap shot. I also had one power-play goal, two power-play points, one shorthanded goal, two game-winning goals, 134 shots on net, and a 14.93 shooting percentage. Overall, it was a good year.

We played Detroit in the division semifinals and won the opening game 9–5. I scored two goals—the first time I had scored two goals in a game the whole season—and felt like it was another sign. I thought to myself, okay, let's get married.

The first goal came on a backhand after a feed from Fras, the other on a slap shot from just inside the blueline. After the first goal, I crashed into the boards and a Wings player skated by me and nicked the back of my helmet. I didn't know if it was accidental or on purpose.

We won the second game 6–1 and swept the series with an 8–2 win in Game 3. I had a goal in the third game and had five points in the series. Fraz had goals in the first two games and three points. Troy had three assists.

We then played Minnesota and beat them in six games. They won the first game 8–5, we won the next three (6–2, 5–3, and 7–6 in double overtime), Minnesota won the fifth game 5–4 in overtime, and we wrapped it up 6–5 in double overtime in their building. Darryl Sutter scored the winning goal. I had two goals and two assists in the series. Troy had two goals and six assists. Fraz had three goals and two assists.

Now we were on to the conference finals against Edmonton, the defending Stanley Cup champions. They had beaten us three times in the regular season—4–2, 6–4, and 7–3. For some players who had been part of the team swept by the Oilers two seasons earlier, this was a painful reminder of something they didn't wish to repeat. Because I was new to the team and hadn't experienced that, I couldn't specifically relate to it, but as someone who had grown up in Chicago and cheered for the Hawks, I understood how deflating that series loss was. Now I was about to experience playing the Oilers in my rookie year with a trip to the Stanley Cup Final on the line.

We were feeling pretty good about our chances going into the series because it was a clean slate. Edmonton hammered us 11–2 in the first game and 7–3 in the second game, but Pully didn't say anything remotely close to what Orval had said. We came home and in the third game some fans displayed a sign that read EDMONTON HAS GRETZKY, BUT CHICAGO HAS FANS.

As I was skating around prior to the anthem, I made eye contact with somebody in the crowd. As I skated by him, I realized it was Chicago Bears running back Gale Sayers. Forget about being one the greatest players in National Football League history; he's one of the greatest athletes of all time. As I skated by him again, he was clapping. I thought, this must be a really important game if Gale Sayers is here.

The crowd was going crazy. It was the loudest I've ever heard it. When Wayne Messmer started signing the Canadian anthem, some of the crowd started booing. There had been some talk that during the games in Edmonton the fans were booing the American anthem. Before Wayne began the first note for the American anthem, the crowd cheered throughout. We won 5–2.

We won the fourth game 8–6 and I scored a shorthanded goal, going around Paul Coffey—Pat Foley said I "was busting through the middle of the ice"—with a slap shot from about 45 feet away, right on the ice, on Grant Fuhr. I heard afterward Pat exclaimed, "And even Coffey couldn't stay with him!" For the record, Paul Coffey is a Hockey Hall of Famer and one of the best skaters to ever play in the NHL, so I'll take that compliment. They still play that highlight occasionally at the United Center. Got lucky, for sure.

Edmonton won 10–5 in the fifth game and ended it 8–2 in the sixth game in our building. It is still the most goals scored by two teams in a six-game series in NHL history.

As an 18-year-old rookie, it was out of control playing in that series and coming within two wins of getting into the Stanley Cup Final. While we were dejected, the pain of losing slowly subsided. The Oilers were a dynasty that would win five Stanley Cups in seven years.

It had been an amazing first season for me in the NHL and I couldn't wait for next year. I didn't know at the time how difficult it would be to make it to a Final. Because I was a rookie and young, I thought we'd make it to the Cup the next season.

* * *

My second season I scored 29 goals and 50 assists and finished third overall in team scoring behind Denis Savard, who had 116 points, and Troy, who had 99. He also won the Frank Selke Trophy awarded annually to the forward who demonstrates the most skill in the defensive component of the game. I scored eight power-play goals and 22 power-play points. I had 218 shots on goal, compared to 134 in my rookie year.

We finished first in the Norris Division with 39 wins in 80 games and 86 points, one more than Minnesota. We faced Toronto in the opening round and felt good about our chances because the Leafs had finished with just 57 points. We opened at home and the Leafs won 5–3. We played the next night and despite leading 4–2, with Denis Savard scoring all our goals, we lost 6–4.

Two days later in Toronto, the Leafs led 5–0 en route to a 7–2 score and the series was over.

Considering the year before, where we were two wins away from getting to the Stanley Cup Final, obviously it was a huge letdown and disappointing. It was a great regular season and we just laid an egg in the playoffs. As a young player getting so close to the Stanley Cup and the next year you're out of the playoffs in the blink of an eye in the first round, you're in shock. I was stunned more than anything else.

CHAPTER 6

HEADING NORTH

AT THE END OF my second season, I decided to buy a townhouse. I had saved some money living at home and at 21 years old, it was time to move out.

Before the 1987–88 season started, the Hawks signed Toronto defensemen Gary Nylund via free agency and the Leafs wanted me as compensation. The Hawks offered center Ken Yaremchuk and defenseman Jerome Dupont, and if the two sides couldn't work out a deal, it would be left up to arbitration judge Edward Houston to decide.

I first became aware of it from Ricky Curran, who told me what was happening. My initial reaction was, "Can this really happen? I'm going to get sent to Toronto for Gary Nylund but it's not a trade, it's compensation?" I didn't know what to think, but that's when I started to learn that professional hockey is a business.

I had a good first season and a really good second season, so being traded was the furthest thing from my mind. Even though Toronto had asked for me in compensation, I was assured by Bill and Ricky that it was going to work itself out and I wasn't going anywhere. In the end, the arbitrator ruled in favor of the Hawks' offer.

My third season started off in the worst possible way before it even began. Early in September, a week before training camp, a friend of mine, Vince Nieland, died in a pool accident while going to school in Arizona.

He was a defenseman and we had played three years together, winning the Midget Nationals in 1982 for Team Illinois. When you play baseball and hockey with guys year-round, you develop friendships and we had remained close.

His death shook up a lot of us. I had never gone through anything like that, experiencing the death of a young person. It was very emotional. You're asking yourself, how and why does something like this happen? I was a pallbearer at his funeral and that's rough stuff for a 20-year-old. Vince was a terrific kid and had great parents, Mr. and Mrs. N, and a wonderful sister, Nadine. We named our second son, Thomas Vincent, in Vince's honor.

I was not in a good place mentally when the season started and I just couldn't get over it. It was just a bad year. I'm not making excuses, but losing a friend like that and going to see his mom and his dad and his sister to pay my respects was just so hard.

When you disappoint in the playoffs the season before, changes are going to happen. That's just the reality. I played wing on the Clydesdales Line but also played some center that year with Al Secord and Mark LaVarre, another Chicago-born player. I didn't score a point until the fourth game, and in the first 10 games I had only one goal, although I had six assists. After 20 games, I had three goals and 11 assists. After 40 games, I had six goals and 19 assists. Overall, we were struggling with a record of 15–19–6. I was not good.

Another thing that changed that season was I had started fighting more. We had toughness all the way through the lineup that season with the likes of Behn Wilson, Curt Fraser, Al Secord, Dave Manson, and Gary Nylund. Overall, by season's end we had seven players totaling 100 or more penalty minutes. I totaled 119 penalty minutes—the most of my career and the only time I exceeded 100 in a season. In a game against Detroit, I totaled 27 penalty minutes. The game before, against Toronto, I had 12 penalty minutes. I had 10 or more penalty minutes five times that season. I was frustrated because of my season and tried to do whatever I could to get involved, including getting in fights. It was a rough year. The fans were getting on me and on the team. It was not an easy situation. All of us were trying, we just weren't getting results.

RICKY OLCZYK
Eddie's brother
It was a difficult time for him and for my parents, too. We heard the rants from the crowd and we didn't respond. We just sat there. We were there to support him and support the Hawks.

We finished the regular season third in the Norris Division with 72 points and got swept by Detroit in the division semifinals. I had a goal and an assist in the series.

I was chosen to play for Team USA that fall in the Canada Cup, a six-country format that also included Canada, the Soviet Union, Sweden, Czechoslovakia, and Finland. It took place between August 28 and September 15 in various Canadian cities and Hartford, where our team was based. Our coach was Badger Bob Johnson.

After opening with wins over Finland and Sweden, we subsequently lost to Canada, the Soviet Union, and Czechoslovakia. The game against Canada took place in Hamilton's Copps Coliseum and drew a sold-out crowd of 17,026. Mario Lemieux scored all of Canada's goals, while Pat LaFontaine and Corey Millen scored our goals.

We returned to Hartford and I was in my room with Bob Mason, whom the Hawks had signed as a free agent away from Washington. There were rumors in the newspapers that I might be dealt. I had heard through Bill Watters and Ricky Curran that the Hawks were looking to make a big move and shake up the team after two years of disappointments. We were watching an episode of *I Dream of Jeannie* and I told Bob I wouldn't be surprised if he ended up living in my house if I got traded.

A few minutes later, I received a call from Bob Pulford informing me I'd be traded along with Al Secord to the Leafs for their former captain Rick Vaive, Steve Thomas, and Bob McGill.

Look, I was disappointed. I was crushed. It doesn't make you feel good when you get traded for the first time, especially having played for your hometown and feeling like you've let everybody down. But then I thought about playing for the Toronto Maple Leafs and what a great opportunity it was—and by the way, I was playing in the Canada Cup, the greatest hockey tournament going on at the time, and I had two games to go and we were still in playoff contention. We ended up losing the last two games.

I didn't know if Chicago had any other trades in the hopper, but once it happened I figured the Leafs must really want me because they tried to get me in the Gary Nylund deal. Chicago wanted to do something to shake things up and Toronto wanted to do the same thing. The Leafs had finished two points behind us in the Norris Division and made it to the division finals, losing to Detroit in seven games.

I immediately called my folks, Bill and Ricky, and Troy Murray. My folks were disappointed, but on the positive side at least another team wanted me.

The Hockey News wrote a story about the trade indicating a handful of my Chicago teammates would be happy to see me go, but a handful would be sorry to see me leave. Of the latter group, my opinion was those were the guys who liked me for being Eddie Olczyk the hockey player and the person, not Eddie Olczyk the kid from Chicago.

It was news when the Hawks drafted me because a kid from Chicago had never been selected in the first round. To be the first one to have that happen came with a lot of attention. I know there was a lot of envy from some of the guys on the team who weren't overly thrilled with the opportunities that came my way as a rookie and the attention I was getting, but I wasn't looking for any of that. I was just looking to play the game of hockey, help the team win games, and win a Stanley Cup for Chicago, which had last won it in 1961. I was always going to be the hometown kid, but I tried to be the best teammate I could.

CURT FRASER
Eddie's teammate

There was so much pressure on Eddie being the golden child from Chicago and playing for the Blackhawks, and sometimes that puts undue pressure on you to perform. When Eddie was traded after his third season, maybe it was better for him because that hometown pressure got relieved a little bit.

It was time to move on and get ready to play. Because I was accommodating to the media and the fans, sometimes you are just put there in that spot without having a say in it. Maybe it was a distraction, I don't know, but it wasn't a distraction my first year and it wasn't a distraction in the second year in our regular season. I had a bad third year and they decided to make a change.

Pully was quoted in the Chicago media as saying this was the most difficult trade he'd ever made.

"Eddie is a Chicago boy I've known for a long, long time, but we needed to make some changes on our team, especially on our right side," he said. "We feel we've gotten some quality players in Vaive and Thomas, and McGill who can give us a little toughness on our back line. In order to do that, we had to give up two quality players in Secord and Olczyk."

Pully was a big supporter of mine since I was 13 years old and he gave me an opportunity to fulfill a dream and play for the Hawks and had supported me through USA Hockey and the Olympic team. He made the trade because he felt in was in the best interest of the team, but he was confident I would do well in Toronto, a franchise he knew well having played there from 1956 through to the end of 1970.

I knew how big the Leafs were in Toronto because I played in Stratford as a 16-year-old, which was close enough to the big city to understand how important the Leafs are. I understood the history, the pressure, and everything that came with representing the Maple Leafs, both on and off the ice. I knew I was going into a hockey hotbed and could not wait for the experience.

CHAPTER 7

LIFE AS A LEAF

PLAYING IN A BUILDING with as much tradition as Maple Leaf Gardens was a big deal. Putting on that Maple Leafs sweater for the first time was like the feeling I experienced putting on the Hawks jersey for the first time. It was an honor and a privilege playing for a team that had had so many great players. It felt like there was some responsibility both on and off the ice.

While I had been told I'd be playing center at some point in Toronto, I began playing right wing on a line with center Russ Courtnall and left wing Wendel Clark.

There was one moment before the season started that I will never forget. We stretched as a team and on the morning of our final preseason game, some of the guys decided to do something really different. A Jane Fonda–like instructor hired by the Leafs was to lead the sessions, but a few of the boys told the instructor to call in sick for the final stretch and we would send a replacement for her. The boys paid her off not to come in—something like $300.

The replacement instructor was a tad late and made a grand entrance wearing an overcoat. Off came the coat and you never saw so many guys ready to stretch and standing at attention. She was an exotic dancer, but that was unbeknownst to many of us. Some of the veterans on the team had been to a strip joint the night before and paid one of the dancers to lead the stretching exercises the next morning. After beginning the exercises, she asked everyone to pair up and then asked Al "Rocket" Secord to come up and assist her, which had been part of the plan. She then spent a couple of minutes stretching in front of Al. The shit-ass grin on Rocket's face was worth every dollar the guys spent on this prank. Guys were roaring, a bonding moment, for sure. When she finished her exercises with Al, we all cheered loudly.

As Gord Stellick, the Leafs GM, wrote in his hilarious memoir, *Stellicktricity*, it all played out to perfection and Al didn't seem to mind being the "butt" of the joke.

Our coach was John Brophy, a career minor-leaguer who was the basis for Reggie Dunlop, the player-coach portrayed by Paul Newman in the fictional hockey movie *Slap Shot*. Playing for Brophy was interesting. He wasn't much for Xs and Os, more of a motivator, the kind of person who would say, "Let's kick their asses." He was a different kind of guy, super intense.

We opened the season in Chicago. I was really nervous going back home and playing that first game as a visitor, wondering how the fans would react. Yes, the boobirds were out. Again, I did not ask to be traded. It was strange and I was kind of glad to get it out of the way right away. We ended up winning 7–5; I didn't factor in the scoring and had a two-minute penalty. Al Secord and Bob McGill got into a fight in the first period.

I scored my first goal in the fourth game of the season and had three in the first 10 games. I also had six assists. I had my best game of the season in the 11th game, scoring a goal and adding five assists in a victory over Winnipeg at home. A six-point game, not bad.

I was eventually moved to center playing with Mark Osborne and Al Secord. In a game against Vancouver in which we were down 5–3, the three of us scored consecutive goals. The game ended 7–7. I also had three assists in the game. In the next 10 games I scored eight goals and had five assists.

All and all, I was feeling a lot less pressure playing in Toronto than in Chicago. I was just playing, not worried about anything, controlling what I could. I was playing in all situations, and even if I had a tough night I was going back on the ice, which is a great feeling for any player. Most importantly, I was proving to myself I could play in the show and produce.

Maple Leaf Gardens had its own character. It was a really special place. Whereas in Chicago you climbed up and down steps to get to and from the dressing room, in Toronto the walk from the dressing room to the bench could mean navigating your way around usherettes or fans going to their seats. It wasn't unusual for people to walk behind the coach on their way to their seats. Beside the bench was a stool behind the door to accommodate an extra body, giving us a little bit more room. It was clogged up enough on the bench because of seats in the crowd that were so close on either side. I liked to sit on the stool and sometimes you'd have to stand up and move out of the way when people would walk right in between me and the ice with popcorn or a pretzel or whatever, and it was like, "Hey, how's it going?" Or you would see a young Leafs fan and give them a high-five or tap them on the head. That's how it was at the Gardens, which was built by Conn Smythe, who owned the team from 1927 to 1961. Harold Ballard, who took over control of the Leafs and Maple Leaf Gardens in 1972, was a master at selling out the building and using every available space to put in seats.

In Chicago, I never had much interaction with owner Bill Wirtz. But he and his family always treated me incredibly well. In Toronto, Mr. Ballard was around all the time and he had a Bouvier dog, TC Puck, who used to fly around the locker room. Mr. Ballard would watch practice from the stands and yell down to Brophy, making sure everyone was listening to him. It was like the voice of God the way he'd yell, "John, John, are the boys listening to you?" Brophy would blow the whistle and bang his stick a couple of times and everything would stop and John would say something like, "Yes, Mr. Ballard."

Mr. Ballard watched the home games in his private box called the Bunker in one end of the arena, a few levels up from the ice. The TV cameras always focused on him because that's the type of presence he commanded. He treated me with full respect and was incredibly friendly to me and my family.

Brophy was not about tender loving care, by any stretch. Whatever he felt, he told you. It didn't matter where you were from or if you understood English or not, whether you were a tough guy or a skill guy. He'd let you know what he was thinking. But he gave me an opportunity to play a lot and I'll be forever grateful for that. I know that I wasn't his type of player—he would probably rather have 20 tough guys than 20 skill guys—but I think he realized if he was going to have a job and win, he needed all types of players. He appreciated what I could and couldn't do. We had our battles and run-ins, but I think I performed well for him.

There was a game in Minnesota against the North Stars at the old Met Center in which we fell behind in the first period. We were sitting in the dressing room at the end of the period wondering if Brophy was going to come into the room and snap because of how badly we played. During intermissions back in the day, guys did a lot of stuff—tape sticks, hydrate, light a dart (cigarette, in hockey parlance), go to the bathroom, see the trainers, or check Twitter (okay, just kidding—there was no such thing as social media back then).

Sure enough, the dressing room door flew open and here came Brophy, ready to go into snap city, F-bombs released every three words. He zeroed in on Al Iafrate.

"Where are you, Iafrate?" he shouted. "Iafrate! Iafrate!"

Al was not in the room. He would usually go into the bathroom stall and light a dart for a few minutes during intermissions. Brophy went into the bathroom and pounded on the stall door.

"Iafrate!" he shouted.

No response, all you heard was a toilet flush.

Out came Al and the boys were biting their lips. Al walked from the bathroom to his locker, shirt off, pants off, skates on. Al is a huge man, 6-foot-4, 230 pounds. Brophy was leaning over Al, who was looking down at the floor, right hand on head, playing with his thinning hair.

"Iafrate, if [5-foot-8] Dennis Maruk is gonna skate by you, the next time take your stick and break his arms. Do you you hear me, Iafrate?"

As he was saying this, Brophy takes a stick to make his point.

No response from Al, who was just staring at the floor with Broph in his space.

Brophy continued screaming at Iafrate and Al was still not responding, and then Broph looked at the top of Al's head.

"Iafrate, you suck, you suck. You're bald. You're bald. You're bald."

I lost it and buried my head in a towel because it was so funny. I wasn't alone. The guys pissed themselves, thinking, this is the NHL? Hilarious. Al did not suck. He was a really good player, but Broph was so mad that Al wouldn't look at him.

On his way out, Brophy said, "That first period it looked like we played like we were asleep out there, so when you sleep, you turn off the lights."

He then hit the light switch and all the lights in the dressing room went out and it was pitch black. The only light was the one coming from the bottom of the door Brophy just went out. It was about 25 seconds until the lights went on. The King, Borje Salming, turned them on. Just as Borje sat down, the door opened and here came Brophy again.

"Who turned on the lights?"

Crickets.

"Was that you, Salming?" Broph asked, throwing in a couple of F-bombs. "Was that you, you chickenshit Swede?"

For the record, Borje Salming was one of the toughest players I ever played with, tough as nails.

Brophy just had a way with words. I don't think he meant it. We finished the game (with the lights on), but lost 4–2. That's the night the lights went out in Minny.

After the game, Brophy lost it when talking to two Toronto reporters, Mark Harding and Lance Hornby, about how we played. He said the F-word 57 times in a rant that was recorded by the reporters. It lasted six minutes and two seconds. After the reporters left to talk to us, Brophy had assistant coach Garry Lariviere call them back because he had more to say.

I finished the season with 42 goals, which ended up becoming a career high, and 75 points. We finished fourth in the Norris Division with 52 points and played Detroit, which finished first with 93 points, in the opening round.

The series opened in Detroit and we won 6–2. The next night they beat us 6–2 and the series shifted to Maple Leaf Gardens. They won 6–3 and two nights later shellacked us 8–0. It would go down as one of the worst playoff defeats in Leafs history. The fans were incensed with how we played—throwing cups, jerseys, pucks, and hats with the words BROPHY'S BOYS on them onto the ice. The fans were frustrated. We were as well. It was disappointing to say the least, but to see some fans acting like that, I was surprised. It was embarrassing.

Two nights later in Detroit we won 6–5 in overtime and I scored a hat trick, including the game-winner 34 seconds into the first OT. It was the first hat trick of my pro career.

One of the reporters asked me what I thought the reaction would be like when we came back to Toronto and I said they should be throwing roses instead of garbage. Sure enough, there were dozens of roses sent to the arena that next day, simply addressed to Eddie and the Leafs.

The fans believed again.

In the warmup before the sixth game, people threw long stem roses on to the ice. But we ended up losing the game 5–3 and the series.

* * *

On August 6, Diana and I married in her hometown of Columbus, Indiana. As a side note, Diana's mother and father, June Ann and Thomas Vickers, were best friends with Ed and Nancy Pence. Of course, the name Pence would become famous worldwide in 2016 as Michael, their son, would become the vice president of the United States. Shortly before Michael became vice president, Diana's mom passed away. Michael and his entire family were all there to support their lifelong family friends.

It was a great wedding. I think there were about 350 people there. We went to Maui on our honeymoon, albeit from Chicago to Toronto, Toronto to San Francisco, and San Francisco to Maui. I think we used the tickets that the team gave us for Christmas. Why not? They were free plane tickets. We bought a home in the north end of the city in Unionville.

Things were about to change significantly for me professionally as well. Russ Courtnall had fallen into disfavor with Brophy, who wanted more toughness in the lineup, and Courtnall would soon be traded. I was placed on a line centering Mark Osborne on left wing and Gary Leeman on right wing. Immediately our line began to click. Ozzie and Gary were great linemates on and off the ice.

I had three goals and four assists after the first three games, which included 7–4 and 8–4 wins over Chicago. After 10 games, we had a record of 6–3–1 and I had six goals and six assists. Gary had six goals and 10 assists. Ozzie had two goals and six assists. We were playing on the power play and also killing penalties. We were dubbed the GEM Line. Every time we stepped on the ice, we felt we would score. Ozzie did the heavy lifting, Gary was the scorer, and I did the facilitating. Our line had it all and we all enjoyed being together on and off the ice. Gary and I carpooled a lot and Ozzie and I roomed together and sat on the plane together in the exit row. He would read the Holy Bible and I would read the horse racing bible, the *Daily Racing Form*. I thought it was a very safe row.

Things were looking good, but we won only three of our next 10 games and had a record of 9–10–1 after 20 games. Things didn't improve much after that. We won only two games in our next 10, losing seven and tying one. During that span, we lost back-to-back games to Minnesota and rumors started to circulate that Brophy would be fired.

On December 1, our first game after the two losses to Minnesota, we played a game in Los Angeles and Brophy cut his head after he hit a steel girder taking a short cut under the stands toward the bench for the third period rather than walking along the ice. In a story headlined "Brophy Bloodied but Not Beaten—Yet," *Toronto Star* reporter Rick Matsumoto wrote that Brophy shooed away trainers and referee Ron Hoggarth when they inquired about his well-being because of the cut. "As the blood turned his snow-white hair crimson red and dropped down on to the shoulder of his gray suit, he dabbed at the wound with a towel," Matsumoto wrote.

We lost the game 9–3 and Brophy needed seven stitches afterward to close the cut. I remember him getting medical attention in the hallway, making sure that all of us could see and hear him.

"C'mon, Doc, I am tough. I am not a chickenshit like these guys. I don't need a Novocain," he said.

That's the legend of Brophy.

On December 19, the day we were to play St. Louis at home, Brophy was fired and replaced on an interim basis by assistant general manager/scout George Armstrong, one of the greatest Leafs of all time. Chief came in and addressed us that morning and said, "Guys, I really don't want to be here, but if I want to get paid…well, here I am." The story goes that George didn't want the job, but Mr. Ballard threatened to fire him if he didn't agree to do it. We had a record of 11–20–2 at the time.

We beat the Blues that night, 4–3. We played in Quebec on December 29 and Gary and I set a team record and tied an NHL record for the fastest two goals in a row by one team. I scored the goal that preceded his and we won 6–5. We closed out the year two days later at home beating

Quebec 6–1 to raise our record to 14–23–2. George delegated most of the duties to assistant coach Garry Lariviere.

Toward the end of the season, Bob Stellick, Toronto's director of communications, nominated me for the NHL's Man of the Year award, pointing out my production on the ice and my charity work as honorary president of the Ontario Special Olympics. He concluded by saying that "as a team without a captain, many consider Ed a player worthy of that distinction."

We had a record of 17–26–4 with Chief and finished the season with a record of 28–46–6, last in the Norris Division.

I finished with 38 goals and 52 assists for a total of 90 points, which would become a career best for me. Gary had 32 goals and 43 assists, both personal bests, and Ozzie had 16 goals and 30 assists.

* * *

On June 17, 1989, Diana and I celebrated the birth of our first child, whom we named Edward Thomas. I was named after my father and out of respect I named our son after him. But we called him Eddie. We didn't know ahead of time if it would be a boy or a girl and asked the doctor not to tell us. We had talked about names for either. I suggested Diana because that was my mom's name and my wife's name.

"How great would that be?" I said.

Diana looked at me the same way she does when I say something off the wall and said, "No, that's not happening."

Alexandra was another name we considered—and would in fact use for our third child.

When you bring a child into this world, it's the most incredible time you can have with your significant other. Everything just stops. You don't know where you are, what city you are in, what your job is. You ask yourself if you're really ready for it. It's just you in your own world and you welcome this human and it's like, "Here's our responsibility. This is us, connected in the best way possible." It's just incredible and really emotional. Diana said having a baby is like an out-of-body experience. It's everything you hear about from other people who have had children but even more so because it is your own child.

Diana likes to collect things and while in Toronto she came across a little plaque that said WE INTERRUPT THIS FAMILY FOR HOCKEY. It became something we hung in our home since that day.

Gary and I became partners that summer owning thoroughbreds, something in which we both had an interest. Gary played for a minor hockey team called Hawley's Horses, sponsored by Hall of Fame jockey Sandy Hawley and the Ontario Jockey Club. Through Ontario Jockey Club publicity director Bruce Walker, who was a friend of Gary's father, we were told about a young, up-and-coming trainer, Mike Mattine. His father, Tony, was a seasoned veteran, particularly good with young horses. I was making $105,000, so it wasn't like I had money to throw around.

In my rookie year with the Blackhawks, I was part of a group that owned a standardbred horse named The Gift Goes On. Denis Savard, my buddy Joe "The Judge" Casciato, Dr. Paul Ruck (the timekeeper for many years at the old Chicago Stadium), and a few others were partners. It cost each of us $3,500 to get in and we bought the horse out of a $25,000 claiming race.

The horse raced for the first time for our group about five weeks later. While we were playing, I got a penalty and went into the penalty box, and Dr. Ruck told me the horse won and paid $50. I couldn't believe it. It had started furthest out in the field and the chances of winning were slim. We didn't go much further in ownership after that. It was the only time the horse won—I didn't even have a win bet—and it was just to have some fun. The horse ended up with a lifetime record of two wins in 29 starts and earnings of less than $8,000.

Gary and I called ourselves the I'm Telling U Stable, the U being an inverted horseshoe. We let Mike decide on the horse we would claim, and the first one he chose was a filly name Regal Rivage, whom he thought he could improve by making some changes. She was a daughter of Vice Regent, whose sire was the great Northern Dancer. We put in the claim slip for $12,500 before the race and were owners of our first horse afterward.

Regal Rivage didn't run particularly well in the race, and afterward Mike had us come back to the barn. He pointed out how her ribs were showing and then he put her on a weight scale. He wanted to put at least 100 pounds on her. Two starts after we claimed her, she won. It was exhilarating to claim a horse, watch it train, see Mike make some improvements, and the next thing you know we're in the winner's circle.

I always seemed to get more worked up when one of my horses was running than anytime I was playing in a hockey game because you have no control over it. You're just hoping the horse has a good trip and doesn't get held up or interfered with or cause interference. Add in the fact I like to bet and have a few tickets in my pocket, well, it's a pretty special time. We also claimed a horse called Mr. Bow Tie and had really good success with him. He was an awesome horse.

The one thing I have always liked about the track is going in the mornings to watch the horses train and talking to people. The backstretch of the track is always filled with lots of characters. I find it peaceful. Whether I have horses training or walking or learning to break from the gate, I've always wanted to be out there.

* * *

The Leafs made two significant changes in hockey operations after the season, hiring Floyd Smith as general manager and Doug Carpenter as head coach. They also acquired defenseman Rob Ramage from Calgary for a second-round pick in the 1989 draft. Smith had a lengthy career as a player in the NHL, from 1954 to 1972, playing for five teams, including the Leafs. He also had a lengthy coaching career. He had been the head coach of the Buffalo Sabres from 1971–72 to 1976–77. In the 1974–75 season, he guided the Sabres to the Stanley Cup Final, losing to Philadelphia. He later coached in the World Hockey Association and for part of the 1979–80 season with the Leafs before he was injured in a car accident. He had been a scout with the team when promoted to GM. Carpenter had been the head coach of the Leafs' farm team in St. Catharines the previous season and had been a head coach with New Jersey from 1984–85 through midway of the 1987–88 season. The Devils did not qualify for the playoffs during his tenure.

Ramage had just won the Stanley Cup with the Flames and was chosen as our captain by Mr. Ballard, who had never even met him. When asked by the media about it, Ballard said, "I'll tell him when I see him."

In November, stories surfaced in the media that I was unhappy with my role because I was not receiving as much ice time as the previous season and wasn't being used on the power play. My numbers from the previous two years were really good, so along with the fans and the media I was wondering what the hell was going on. I respected Doug, but it just seemed like whenever I turned left, he thought I should have turned right.

Carpenter had us playing on the third line and alternated Wendel Clark with Ozzie. I had five goals and seven assists in 15 games in which the team had a 6–9 record and I made it known in the media I wasn't happy with the situation. I was asked a few questions and I answered them. While there had been rumors I was on the trade block, Smith denied that when asked by the media. Carpenter told the media that it was a "cop-out" for me suggesting the team was trying to trade me.

We won four of our next five and I scored three goals and added three assists. Things started to improve for the team and me in the next 20 games. We had a record of 18–21–1. In 18 straight games between December 2 and January 8, I had at least a point a game, trying a Maple Leafs scoring record set by the great Darryl Sittler and setting an NHL record for an American-born player. During the streak I had 11 goals and 17 assists and our record was 10–7–1.

We started to put it together in the final 40 games, posting a record of 20–17–3 to finish with an overall record of 38–38–4, third in our division. It proved to be a great year for myself, Gary, and Ozzie. I finished with 32 goals and 56 assists, which became a career high, and 88 points, only two shy of my season before. Gary scored 51 goals, only the second player in Leafs history to surpass the 50-goal mark, an increase of 19 from the year before, and totaled a career-best 95 points. Ozzie had 23 goals, a career-best 50 assists, and a career-best 73 points, 27 more than the previous year. Gary had 14 power-play goals, I had six, and Mark had three. We became the highest-scoring line in team history. Can you imagine the numbers we might have had if the coach had played us together a little more earlier in the season? I still do.

We played St. Louis, which finished second in the division with three more points, in the opening round of the playoffs. St. Louis won the first two games, each with a 4–2 score. We returned home and lost Game 3 6–5 in overtime. We rebounded to win the next game 4–2. The next day Mr. Ballard, who was in the hospital and in extremely poor health, died at the age of 86.

We played Game 5 the next day and lost 4–3.

Gary led the team with three goals, two of them on the power play, and three assists. Ozzie was next with two goals and three assists. I had a goal and two assists.

* * *

Diana and I were expecting our second child in November, so this was an exciting time for us. We didn't know whether the child would be a boy or a girl, only that the birth would happen in Toronto, similar to what took place with Eddie the previous June. This was another indication about how much the city meant to us. Toronto had become our home.

Physically and mentally, I was gearing up for the start of the 1990–91 season and looking forward for the team to improve and for our line to follow up on the success we just had. Both Gary and Ozzie were also excited about the upcoming season.

We started out with a three-game road trip out west, losing 7–1 to Winnipeg, 4–1 to Calgary, and 3–2 to Edmonton. I scored my first goal of the season in the Oilers game. We weren't a great defensive team, but the year before we found a way to score. If we gave up five, we'd score six. If we gave up six, we'd score eight. That's how we played. Did we help our goalies? No. We knew what our strengths and weaknesses were, but when you're not scoring and you're not good defensively, that's not a good combination.

Playing for the Leafs was never an issue until the fourth year. For some reason, my ice time diminished from the season before. It was like management was saying, "We have a plan and you're not going to be part of it." So after having scored 42, 38, and 35 goals, respectively, the three previous seasons, I wasn't being played as much.

We had our home opener against Quebec and lost 8–5. I had three assists, all on the power play. In the fifth game, we tied Detroit at home 3–3, recording our first point of the season. Following losses to Hartford and Chicago, in which we were outscored 6–1, we finally won our first game of the season, beating the Blackhawks 6–2 at home. We then began another losing streak, starting with a 5–1 defeat on the road to the New York Rangers, 8–3 to St. Louis at home, and 8–5 to the Blues in St. Louis. Gary scored his second goal of the season and I assisted on it.

We were 1–9–1 after 11 games and that's when Floyd Smith decided to fire Carpenter. It's inevitable when you get off to such a bad start, something's going to happen. There was some speculation of a big trade or the coach getting whacked.

Tom Watt, who had been a head coach of Winnipeg and Vancouver and had been hired as Carpenter's assistant in the off-season, was promoted to replace him. I really didn't know much about him prior to his joining the Leafs. I was hoping it would be a new lease on life for me. As a player, the first thing you are thinking about when a new coach comes in is how it is going to going to affect you. Do I have a relationship with the new coach? Am I a part of what's moving forward? If you have a relationship with a guy and you like him and he likes you, you're in like Flynn.

I had only one goal at that point, Gary had two, and Ozzie had three. Collectively we were having a hard time generating the kind of offense we enjoyed the season before.

We lost 3–1 at home to Buffalo in our first game with Watt and then defeated Minnesota 5–4 two nights later at home. But the euphoria didn't last long. We followed up with a five-game losing streak and were outscored 28–14. You knew player changes were coming because our record was brutal. I had talked to my agents, Billy Watters and Rick Curran, because they had heard some rumors and speculation I might be traded, but nothing was imminent as far as they knew. All I could do was read the newspapers and watch TV for some information.

On November 9, the Leafs made two moves, acquiring center Mike Krushelnyski from Los Angeles and winger Rob Cimetta from Boston. Meanwhile, later that night, Diana went into labor.

I called Bob Stellick and let him know I wouldn't be at practice the next morning but planned to play in the game that night against Chicago because Diana would have delivered the baby by then. The game was going to be televised on *Hockey Night in Canada* at 8:00 PM. I also called Ozzie and Gary because I wanted them to know Diana had gone into labor.

The next morning, I called Bob again to say Diana hadn't delivered the baby yet, but we expected it to happen soon and I planned to play in the game.

Diana was starting to dilate at about 4:00 PM and the obstetrician said, "Let me put my catcher's mitt on." At about 4:15, a nurse came into the delivery room and handed me a note that said the Maple Leafs were on the phone. I told her to tell them Diana was having the baby and that I would be at the game.

I turned my attention back to Diana: "Breathe, Diana, you are doing great. Breathe."

The nurse came back 45 seconds later and told me the team really wanted to talk to me. I left the delivery room, but at that time I still had no idea why the team wanted to talk to me. I'm in the middle of waiting for my second child to be born and wasn't thinking about anything else but that. Diana was like six out of 10 on the birthing scale, so, like an idiot, I left the room. When I arrived at the nurses' station and answered the phone, Bob Stellick was on the line.

He's super cool and said, "How's Diana?"

"Bob, she's having the baby. I'll be at the game. I'll see you later," I said.

"No, no, call us before you come."

"I'm not calling you. I can't. I'll be at the game."

"Hold on a second."

Then Floyd Smith was on the line.

"Hey, Floyd, what's up?" I said.

"Eddie, we really hate to do this to you, but we've just traded you to the Winnipeg Jets."

My heart stopped. Seriously?

"You're kidding me," I said.

"No, it's out there and we had to officially tell you."

He added that he gave Jets general manager Mike Smith my information and that I should call him when I got a chance.

I hung up on him and sat there in a haze for 30 seconds, thinking, did they really just call me out of the delivery room to tell me I was traded?

BOB STELLICK
Maple Leafs director of communications
It was awful to make the call telling Eddie he was traded, because Diana was having a baby. I wasn't making the trades. At that point there was no assistant GM to call the players to tell them they were traded. It was assigned as one of my 19 tasks in that wacky year. Everybody liked Eddie. There was never any malice. The trade was the business of hockey—an unfortunate part of the game.

My next thought was, now what?

I went to a pay phone and called Ozzie and Gary. Ozzie was at home eating his pregame meal when he received the call. He and his wife, Madolyn, had been married for a couple of years, and while the trade was shocking they didn't have any children, so they didn't have to deal with that additional stress.

Because Ozzie had been traded twice before and this was the second time for me, we both were experienced in this. But as Ozzie recalls, we never thought it was going to happen again, especially given the previous season. Ozzie says that once you get past the surprise factor, reality sets in and you realize you have no control over it. Then it becomes a matter of trying to pick up the pieces and getting your head on straight to go to your new team.

When a trade is made, it means one team wants your services, so you have to think about it that way instead of one team has just decided it doesn't need you anymore.

I also called my folks and Ricky Curran. Neither my parents nor Ricky knew at that point.

The first thing my dad said was, "How's Diana?" They thought I was calling them to say Diana had given birth.

"She's still in labor," I said, "but I wanted to let you know I've been traded."

He recalled immediately asking, "To Winnipeg?" My dad had played golf a few times at the Olympic tryouts with Mike Smith and recalled he really liked me.

Coincidentally, Winnipeg was playing in Chicago the next night.

DIANA OLCZYK
Eddie's mother

I couldn't believe that they did it that way. What were they thinking? They couldn't care less. You're just a piece of meat.

I blasted the Leafs while talking to Ricky and he told me he felt bad the Leafs traded me while Diana was having a baby instead of waiting. That's when it really hit me this is a business and always will be a business. I signed on the dotted line and I get it, but it wasn't right. To me, it was a lack of respect for me and my family. It's about as disrespectful at you can get. If they had waited two or three hours, absolutely that would have been better, but they chose to do it at that time and that's fine.

On the other hand, I thought, play better and you wouldn't get traded. That's the reality of it. I had only four goals and 10 assists in 18 games.

I was probably gone from the delivery room for five to six minutes, but it felt like half an hour. When I walked back in, the doctor was still in the same position as when I left. Diana looked at the ceiling and then back at me and asked, "Where in the hell have you been?"

I couldn't believe how all of this went down and I didn't want to tell her.

I took a step back and said, "My aunt is sick."

Diana looked away and then looked back at me and said, "Where are we going?"

I said to myself, "Is she really a psychic? Is this what happens when you're giving birth?" A psychic pregnant lady, oh my.

I thought this must be some kind of a game.

"Well, guess?" I said.

She looked at me and then the ceiling again and said, "Winnipeg."

I was stunned. I didn't answer for a few seconds.

She looked at me, and I nodded my head yes.

And then she just shut down and the doctor put his catcher's mitt away for a while. There was no way she was in any condition mentally to give birth. I gave her a hug and talked through everything that had happened. I guess Thomas Olczyk decided to prolong his entry into this world a little longer.

The trade was devastating because I had my three best years in terms of point production in my career at that point. Any time you get uprooted, especially the way it happened, it's tough psychologically. I was emotional because we really loved living in Toronto, but also how it all came apart and how it affected my wife. It was such a private moment when the team decided to make that decision and I took it very personally.

DIANA OLCZYK
Eddie's wife

The way the trade was handled, I guess I kind of look at it and say it was a little bit raw, but what else were they supposed to do? It was a phone call at the nurses' station. Would they have sent someone? I don't know. He had a game that night—would he have shown up at the rink and found out he had been traded and was not playing and left me there? Labor slowed down after that and we joked that Tommy must have known we were going to Winnipeg and he didn't want to go somewhere cold because he liked it where he was. It was nice and warm. In retrospect you could say they could have handled it more professionally.

Ozzie said what happened was typical of the generation in which we played, whereas in today's NHL there is more consideration toward the players from the team. He thought the trade was disappointing and frustrating when you think about the fact the team knew Diana was in labor and still made the deal.

Two and a half hours after I learned I was traded, Tommy Olczyk was born. We had decided if the child was a boy we were going to name him after Diana's father. We had already experienced the miracle of birth once before, and felt as blessed this time around as the first time. Despite all that had happened that day, in that exact moment you put it all aside.

The Leafs lost 5–1 to the Hawks that night and Gary suffered a separated shoulder when he was checked by Hawks forward Mike Hudson. It's crazy how things happened.

I went home, picked up a suit, and flew to Chicago to meet my new team. I was only going to be away for a day because the Jets played the Leafs the following night back in Toronto. Diana wasn't going to be coming home from the hospital until the following Tuesday, so it was time to regroup and focus on hockey. It helped that I was traded with Ozzie.

I was given my No. 16 and walked into the Jets dressing room. I knew some players from international play or having played against them over the years. The hockey community is fairly tight, even though we come from various parts of the world. I told my teammates about being in the delivery room when I found out I was traded and the guys started laughing and talking about it. That's just hockey, and even if that specific situation hasn't happened to a player personally, he can probably relate to it in some way.

Ozzie and I were now Jets and had to focus on the game at hand. We didn't know any of the team's systems, specific line combinations, who played on the power play or killed penalties. We would essentially be playing on our hockey instincts. Even though we were new to the team, it's as if the guys in the room were saying to us, "Grab an oar. You're on our team."

The game ended in a 3–3 tie. Troy Murray, my onetime linemate on the Clydesdales Line, scored two goals for the Hawks.

I saw my parents after the game and we talked for a bit, but then I had to head off for the team bus and go to the airport to fly out to Toronto.

There was a morning skate, and Ozzie remembers how weird it was to come on to the ice from the opposite entrance from where we had normally come out with the Leafs just a few days before. I saw Gary, who was wearing a sling, and we chatted.

GARY LEEMAN
Eddie's teammate

The best line on the team was being broken up. Why would you do that? Why would you trade something that works? Does it surprise me they made the trade when he was in the hospital and Diana was giving birth? How the hell could somebody do that? It just didn't make any sense.

For me, it was disappointing. I was sad and disappointed and I felt terrible for the situation Eddie had to go through with Diana being in labor. Nothing ever made sense in Toronto. The whole thing was a joke. That was just another example of how unprofessional the Toronto Maple Leafs were at that time, trading a guy not knowing he's in the delivery room with his wife.

During one of the intermissions of the Toronto game, I became emotional in a TV interview talking about the trade and how much I was going to miss my former teammates, notably Gary, and the city of Toronto. Diana was still in the hospital and I was speaking from the heart and let it all out. I just wanted a chance to thank the fans. It was an honor wearing that Leafs jersey and I wanted everybody to know that.

We lost the game 5–2. In the second period, with the Leafs leading 2–0, I scored at 5:26 with an assist from Ozzie. I know it felt really good to score a goal even though we got our heads handed to us.

After the game, the Toronto media crowded around me in the dressing room to talk about the trade. I repeated that I loved my time in Toronto because it really helped jump-start my career. After the game I headed back to hospital to visit Diana and Thomas.

From Saturday night through Monday night, I had played games in Chicago and Toronto for my new team and then I was back in the hospital to visit Diana and Tommy. It was pretty crazy the way it all played out.

In my time in Toronto with the Leafs, there were moments when it looked and felt like a circus. In a little more than three years, I had played for four coaches (John Brophy, George Armstrong, Doug Carpenter, and Tom Watt). Some players may not go through that many in their entire careers. The one constant through it all was Mr. Ballard. He was like the forerunner of George Steinbrenner and Jerry Jones. He was a lightning rod, and because it was his team he could do what he wanted.

With the Leafs, I had a chance to play for another NHL Original Six team. And similar to Chicago Stadium, I had a chance to experience one of the oldest and most treasured arenas in hockey. Maple Leaf Gardens had so much history and had been the home to some of the greatest players in NHL history.

But now I was a Winnipeg Jet and had to put all of my memories about Toronto and the Maple Leafs aside. My career was about to go in a new and different direction.

I went back to the hospital, picked up Diana and Tommy, and went home for the day. I packed a suitcase and then flew to Winnipeg on Wednesday for a practice and a game the next day.

CHAPTER 8

A QUESTION OF TIMING

IT WAS EMOTIONALLY HARD being away from Diana and the boys following the trade to the Jets. There is a part of you that sits there and says, "This isn't right." But it's what I signed up for.

Diana always had someone there to help her, whether it was her mom or my mom, and we always had babysitters. We knew once we got our feet set, Diana and the kids would move to Winnipeg. I called every day and sometimes I'd hold the phone two feet away from my ear because Diana needed to vent about being a mom for the second time, with her husband not around and having a 15-month-old boy and a newborn baby. I felt guilty, for sure. It was a sensitive time, but that's why I hurried and found a place to rent in the suburbs and they came in January. Ozzie and I lived in separate rooms in the Country Inn Extended Suites by the Winnipeg airport for the initial period following the trade.

I knew a little bit about Winnipeg because I had gone there for 48 hours for the midget camp of the Winnipeg Warriors of the Western Hockey League in 1981. Winnipeg was also famous because Hawks great Bobby Hull signed with the Winnipeg Jets of the World Hockey Association in 1972.

The Jets had a 7–9–1 record at the time of the trade that brought me to Winnipeg. They were in rebuilding mode after trading center Dale Hawerchuk, the team's captain, in a blockbuster, multi-player deal in June for Buffalo Sabres defenseman Phil Housley. Hawerchuk had played nine seasons in Winnipeg, which had the misfortune of playing in the same division as Edmonton during the Oilers' dynasty in the 1980s. Hawerchuk, whom the Jets selected first overall in the 1981 NHL draft, won Rookie of the Year honors in 1982, totaling 103 points. He surpassed 100 points in six of his first seven seasons.

Housley played eight seasons with the Sabres, who drafted him sixth overall in the 1982 draft. He was on the NHL's All-Rookie Team after totaling 19 goals and 47 assists in 77 games. He had totaled a career-best 81 points in his final year before the trade. He had scored 20 or more goals in five of his eight seasons. Three times he played in the NHL All-Star Game and would do it seven times overall. I had been a teammate of his in the 1984 and 1987 Canada Cup and the 1986 and 1989 World Championships.

Besides Housley, Winnipeg had Randy Carlyle, who had won the Norris Trophy in 1980–81 when he scored 16 goals and 67 assists in 76 games with Pittsburgh. Howie, Randy, Freddy Olausson, and Moe Mantha made for a good defense corps, which is likely the reason the Jets felt they could part with Dave Ellett, who was a really good defenseman.

Thomas Steen, who centered the top line, was appointed captain, taking over from Hawerchuk. Steen was in his 10th season with the team and had totaled 80 points twice, including the 1988–89 season. He would go on to play 14 seasons in the NHL, all with the Jets, and have his jersey No. 25 retired. I considered him one of the most underrated players of my era. His son Alex would hang around the dressing room. Now, all these years later, he's a Stanley Cup champion himself, a member of the 2018–19 St. Louis Blues.

So, my immediate reaction was there were some good players on the team. It was very comfortable, but that's probably because the second time you are traded you have already been through the shock of it, even if this deal was tough because of the circumstances in which it happened.

The whole organization was great, starting with owners Barry and Rena Shenkarow, general manager Mike Smith, and coach Bob Murdoch. They told me whenever I needed to go home to go do it. If I needed to spend an extra day on the road, that was okay, just show up for the games.

I was so sour about what the Leafs had done pulling me out of the delivery room. You could badmouth me and screw me over, but when you start screwing with my family or my kids, that's where the line was crossed.

But now I had gone from one situation where they had shown no respect for my wife or my family to a place where they were there for me for whatever I needed. They wanted to make sure my family was looked after and I'll be forever grateful for that. That was really important to me. I'm a believer that your players and your coaches and your trainers and everybody in the organization should be looked after. Doesn't matter their salary, title, or role. I think that's how you get the ultimate performance from everyone in the organization, whether you're winning or losing.

I don't think the trade showed me another side of the business. It was more like it reassured me that even though it's a business and you play a game, there are people who are compassionate. I'd like to think I have a little compassion myself.

The Jets' attitude helped Diana, too. She was disappointed about how it all went down and had no say about where we were going. No matter where I was traded, it wouldn't have mattered to her.

Winnipeg is a real hockey community. It always has been, whether it was in the World Hockey Association with the Jets, whose stars included Bobby Hull, Anders Hedberg, and Ulf Nilsson, or in the NHL. The people are incredible and the support is off the charts. We always had about 500 people watching our practices, and when I asked Carl the security guard at the building how they managed to get in, he would be like Sergeant Schultz of *Hogan's Heroes* and say, "I know nothing. I see nothing." All I know is at $5 a head, that's a pretty good nothing! Carl was such a great guy.

The Jets have always done incredible work with the community. They really have an impact on the town. It mattered then and it does now, especially when the team was brought back by the NHL in 2011, 15 seasons after it was moved to Phoenix and then re-branded in Atlanta. Mark Chipman has done a great job of bringing the Jets back. The people get so jacked up for the games, painting their faces and wearing the same gear. It's a combination of both the Green Bay Packers and Oklahoma City Thunder, both cities with small populations but incredibly devoted fans. Their team is all that matters to them.

I started to fit in well, centering a line with Ozzie on the left and Paul MacDermid on the right, receiving regular ice time on the power play. It felt great to be used in the way I had in my first three seasons in Toronto.

In December, we had a 10-day road trip starting in Los Angeles, and the day before the first game I went to Hollywood Park with my teammate, Pat Elynuik, who is also a horse guy. I probably had about $1,000 on me, and going over my *Daily Racing Form,* I liked a horse in the third race. It had so much speed in it I thought this horse could win without any problems if it just sat behind the pace. The horse was going off at 9-2 odds, which was a great price. I found another horse that two races previously had come off of the pace and the horse finished really well. The next race the horse was sent to the lead, tired, and finished well back, beaten by 20 lengths. The horse's form looked absolutely awful, but I wondered why they would send the horse to the lead when it runs better coming from behind. The horse was 40-1, which is a real long shot, and I thought it had a heck of a chance to finish second with the way the race set up.

The race unfolded as I expected and the 9-2 horse took the lead and sure enough from the far outside comes the 40-1 shot and I have a $50 exacta with the 9-2 shot over the 40-1 shot. If the horses finish in that order, I'm getting 25 times the payoff. The 9-2 wins and the 40-1 shot finished second. The exacta paid almost $400 and I cashed almost $10,000. What a way to start a 10-day road trip. I was thinking, what am I going to do with this money?

I didn't want to leave the cash in my hotel room or in my pants when we went to practice. The only guys you can trust are the trainers, so the next morning at practice I approached Craig Heisinger, our head equipment manager and now the assistant general manager with the Jets.

"I need a favor from you," I said.

"What do you need?" he asked.

"I need you to hold on to this money."

He always had shorts on, whether it was 40 below or 40 above. Skating by him during practice I'd say, "You're walking a little heavy on that right side." I was referring to the money. For every game during the road trip, I had him hold the money because I didn't want to leave it in the locker room. Every once in a while, during a timeout, I'd ask him, "You all right? You still got the money?" He would just grab his pocket. It's hard not to miss a wad of $10,000 and a guy wearing gym shorts on a hockey bench.

Of course, I took care of Zinger. A great human and a smart guy, too. He always makes me smile and he loves my wife's homemade fudge.

All the guys on the team said they should have given me money to bet. I told them if anyone would have given me $10, I would have brought them back almost $2,000.

When I called Diana, I said I had a good day at the track.

Much was made about the Leafs playing us at home on February 6. Honestly, I don't remember much about that game—so much has happened in my career and life since that time—which finished in a 5–5 tie. But looking at some newspaper clippings, I didn't hesitate to talk about Leafs, who were struggling. In a story written by Lance Hornby of the *Toronto Sun* under the headline "Olczyk Takes Shot at Leafs," I made it clear I was still miffed, and maybe more so because I was still upset about the way the trade was done.

"If people thought that [trade] was going to solve the problem, that the Leafs were suddenly going to go on to bigger and better things, then I guess the games have spoken for themselves," I said. "It's gone the other way. I've learned a lot from that situation, but nobody can ever take away what I accomplished in Toronto, what we did as a team, and what Gary and I had as a friendship."

I was asked about the misconception of my time in Toronto, beginning with my close relationship with Gary and that we were too selfish for the team's welfare.

"That's the kind of thing that bothered me the most—the perception," I said. "You hear it somewhere and it's etched in stone. No one ever said anything about Daniel [Marois] and Vince [Damphousse] hanging out together."

Looking back on the score sheet of the game, I scored a goal and Ozzie had an assist.

With the tie we raised our record to 20–29–9, while the Leafs had a 14–35–6 record.

We went into a slump in the final 20 games, winning only five, which knocked us out of qualifying for the playoffs. We finished with a record of 26–43–11 for a total of 63 points, last in the Smythe Division and ninth in the Campbell Conference, six points ahead of Toronto. Phil Housley led the team in scoring with 76 points in 78 games, followed by Thomas Steen, who had 67 points in 58 games and Pat Elynuik with 65 points in 80 games.

I totaled 26 goals and 31 assists in 61 games, finishing fourth in total points. I had 14 power-play goals and 22 power-play points. I had a point-a-game streak during a stretch of nine games between February 14 against New Jersey and March 5 against Edmonton, totaling seven goals and seven assists.

I decided to change agents around this time. Rick Curran had become busy since Bill Watters left the Branada Sports Management agency to become assistant general manager of the Leafs early in the 1993 season.

Rick became increasingly busier and I decided to hire Ronnie Salcer, who had a smaller agency.

Deciding to leave Rick was very difficult and so hard to do. I really want to thank him for everything he did to help me along this journey. So, why did I choose Ronnie? Here's an example: back when I was 15 years old and had all those agents calling me, as soon as I told them I was going with Rick and Billy, they pretty much hung up on me. I felt they were more interested in what I could do for them than they were in what was best for me and my future. But not Ronnie. He told me, "Those guys are great. If I can ever help you out, let me know. Good luck." That showed me Ronnie cared about me even though it didn't benefit him at the time. I remembered that when it came time to choose a new agent.

In June, the team underwent a significant change when John Paddock replaced Bob Murdoch as coach. This was John's first head coaching job in the NHL. He had coached six seasons in the American Hockey League and won the league championship with the Hershey Bears in 1988.

About a month after the change in coaches, Mike Smith acquired my former Hawks teammate and linemate Troy Murray and Warren Rychel for Bryan Marchment and Chris Norton.

I was selected to be part of the U.S. team in the 1991 Canada Cup, the third time I had been chosen for that tournament, which included Canada, Finland, Sweden, the Soviet Union, and Czechoslovakia. It took place between August 31 and September 16. Our team's general manager, Craig Patrick, publicly declared this would be the best American squad of all time in international play. In addition to me, the team included Doug Brown, Chris Chelios, Dave Christian, Tony Granato, Kevin Hatcher, Brett Hull, Pat Jablonski, Craig Janney, Jim Johnson, Pat LaFontaine, Brian Leetch, Kevin Miller, Mike Modano, Joey Mullen, Joel Otto, Mike Richter, Jeremy Roenick, Gary Suter, John Vanbiesbrouck, Eric Weinrich, Craig Wolanin, and Randy Wood. Our coach was once again Badger Bob Johnson, who was coach of the Pittsburgh Penguins at the time.

We opened with a 6–3 win over Sweden in Toronto. We played Canada in our second game, which took place in Hamilton, and lost 6–3. We won our remaining three round-robin games: 4–2 over Czechoslovakia in Detroit, 2–1 over the Soviet Union in Chicago, and 4–3 over Finland in Chicago. Canada finished with a record of 3–0–2, but was placed ahead of us on the basis of its victory in the round-robin. Finland placed third at 2–2–1, followed by Sweden (2–3–0). We cruised to a 7–3 win over Finland in our semifinal game played in Hamilton, while Canada blanked Sweden 4–0 in Toronto in the other semifinal.

There was a great sense of anticipation about us playing Canada in the final, given how Craig Patrick had built up our team. The best-of-three series opened in Montreal and Canada won 4–1. What will be remembered more than the actual score was an incident in which Gary Suter crosschecked Wayne Gretzky, who was knocked out of the tournament.

Two days later the second game took place in Hamilton. After a scoreless first period, Canada jumped out to a 2–0 lead in the second on goals by Mark Messier and Steve Larmer, but we tied it up with goals by Jeremy Roenick and Kevin Miller. Larmer scored a shorthanded goal at 12:13 of the third period to give the Canadians the lead and Canada added a goal by Dirk Graham to win 4–2.

My focus turned to the 1991–92 season, one during which I ended up playing with a contract that had already expired. You read that right. My agent, Ronnie Salcer, couldn't agree to terms with Jets GM Mike Smith, so we filed for salary arbitration. At that time, the salary arbiter would set the date and in this case, it was set for a year from the time we filed to go arbitration. So, I played that year with the salary from the final year of the expired deal.

What would have happened if I had been injured? I have no idea. That's the way the rules were at the time. It was a loophole for the league and the team to get a one-year deal at the same number before I would go to arbitration. Can you imagine a star player today going to arbitration and being told it couldn't be heard for a year? That was the system back then.

I started off strongly with five goals and three assists in the first 10 games. After 20 games, I had 11 goals and 11 assists. After 30 games, I had 15 goals and 15 assists. After 40 games, I had 19 goals and 24 assists. It was the best season of my career, and I thought for sure I was going to go to my first All-Star Game.

And then my season came to a stop on January 8 in a game against Edmonton in which I scored the winning goal. The Oilers' Craig Simpson was coming down the left side and I was coming from the right-hand side. Simmer got to the top of the circle and cut into the middle to give himself a better angle and I tried to impede his progress with my left arm. He leaned in and I stuck my arm out and got tangled up with him and we ran into our goalie. My right ankle hit the crossbar and I tried to lift my left arm and my elbow was dislocated. It was the worst pain ever.

It was the only time in my career I was carried off on a stretcher and Diana was waiting for me at the end of the ice. I remember telling the first responders in the ambulance to give me something to numb the pain. I had surgery that night to repair the dislocated elbow and walked out of the hospital looking like I'd been in a battle and a half. I was walking with my left arm in a sling and my right foot in a boot and a crutch in my right hand.

I remember on the drive home telling Diana to stop the car on the main thoroughfare and puking everywhere because I was so nauseous. I was also incredibly frustrated. I missed about six weeks, even though I probably should have stayed out longer, but that's what you do when you want to play again. I returned to the lineup for the final 20 games and scored 13 goals and added nine assists.

Of the 32 goals I scored, seven were game-winners and 12 came on the power play. Not a bad season in terms of production, but disappointing nonetheless because of the injury.

Phil Housley led the team with 23 goals and 63 assists for 86 points and placed third in the Norris Trophy voting for top defenseman. Brian Leetch, who was playing for the New York Rangers, won it, scoring 22 goals and 80 assists for 102 points. Two of the greatest American defensemen to ever play in the NHL.

We finished fourth in the Smythe Division with 81 points and faced Vancouver, which led the division with 96 points, in the playoffs. We were third overall in goals allowed with 244 and tied Montreal with seven shutouts. The big difference from the previous season was how much better we did in the final 20 games, winning nine, losing seven, and tying four. We had six wins and two ties in the final eight games.

We were feeling good about ourselves going into the series against Vancouver because of how we finished the season. The series opened in Vancouver and we won 3–2 and I had the game-winner. Vancouver won the second game 3–2. In the third game in Winnipeg, we won 4–2 and then won Game 4, 3–1. We were one win away from winning the series. Vancouver thumped us 8–2 in the Game 5, in which I had one of the goals. We returned to Winnipeg and lost 8–3. In the series' final game, we lost 5–0. It was a disappointing way to go out.

I played in six of the seven games; I missed one game with back spasms, the first time in my career I ever had back issues. It happened in Game 2. All I did was lean over for a faceoff and, bam, it was like a knife in my lower back and I couldn't breathe. It could not have come at a worse time. I finished with two goals and an assist in the series. Thomas Steen and Fredrik Olausson led our team with six points apiece, followed by Phil Housley with five points.

* * *

I remember the 1991–92 season for another reason—I purchased a horse and named her Diana O. as an anniversary present for my wife. I had Mike Mattine's father, Tony, who was an excellent trainer, particularly with young, developing horses, buy the filly in the winter for $32,000 at a two-year-old sale in Florida. I told Tony beforehand I didn't want to spend more than $25,000, but if there was something he liked and it was worth it, he could go higher. It was a Cutlass horse out of a Wancha mare. I knew a little bit about Cutlass as a sire. The filly's mother turned out to be a prolific mare, producing two horses that won $1 million each.

J.R. Smith Sr. trained the horse and he always referred to me as the Hockey Guy. If he had a horse racing and you asked him if he had a shot, he'd look down at you and take the cigar out of his mouth and say, "I entered it, didn't I?" He was a great guy, an incredible trainer, but that was his personality.

Diana O. ran for the first time on September 30 at Arlington Park in Chicago in a 6½-furlong race and won by 4½ lengths, leading the field of 10 all the way. She was second in the odds at just under 4–1 with jockey Jerry La Sala in the irons. We entered her 17 days later at Hawthorne Park in Chicago, this time in a 6-furlong race in a field of six. Jerry rode her again and this time she won by 6¼ lengths. It wasn't a surprise to the bettors, who made her the 3-10 favorite.

We decided to run her next in the $75,000 Pocahontas Stakes, a one-mile race at Churchill Downs in Kentucky on November 1. It was a day before the Breeders' Cup World Championships and we thought about entering her in the $1 million Juvenile Fillies' race, but we thought it was simply too big of a step up and would have cost a lot to enter into it. We all agreed the move was to go into the Pocahontas.

We had talked the night before the race because it was raining and J.R. wanted to know if I still wanted to run the filly. Her sire produced offspring that were monsters on off tracks. I thought she'd love it. J.R. said she loved the off track, so it was a no-brainer to run her. But there was hesitation because of the wet track.

I couldn't attend the race because we had a game at home against Calgary. I went to Grapes Restaurant out by the airport because it had a satellite dish and could bring in the race replay show from Churchill

Downs. In those days there was nowhere to watch it live because there was no simulcasting. So, for me, it was like watching it live and I was really nervous. It was about 4:30 PM Central time and there were only a handful of people at the restaurant and the only person who knew I was there was Diana. Right before the race comes on, I hear "Eddie Olczyk, phone call" over the intercom system at the restaurant. How did anybody know I was there? I get handed the phone and it's Diana calling from home

"Have you seen the race?" she asked.

"No, I'm going to watch it. It's coming up."

"You can't watch it."

"What do you mean?"

"Diana O. broke her leg and they had to put her down."

My heart stopped.

I hung up the phone and went back to the TV.

She said Joe and Dom, who were partners in Diana O. and were at the race, called to tell her what happened. We had hired Gary Stevens because this was a big-time race on a big-time track and I figured we needed a big-time jock. At that time, Gary was one of the top jocks in the country. Diana O. had post five in the field of nine. It was pouring rain during the race and the track was sloppy. Diana O. was fifth in the race after the opening quarter of a mile, about 5 lengths off of the lead. After a half mile, she was fourth by about 2 lengths, and after three quarters she was fourth by 4 lengths. At the top of the stretch she was in sixth place, about 8 lengths back off the lead.

She must have been held up five times to this point but was still full of run. She split horses and an eighth of a mile from the wire she got the lead. At this point I was thinking, we're going to win, she's the real deal, we've got a super filly on our hands. Maybe Joe and Dom were just pulling a prank. The next thing you know, she takes a bad step and broke her right hind leg. Stevens pulled her up and they had to euthanize her.

When I saw it, I lost it. I got so sick, distraught beyond words. It hit me like a ton of bricks. I just couldn't believe it happened. I had turned down an offer from a guy in Florida who wanted to buy her for $250,000 five weeks before that. Even though I was in the sport as an owner for the money, I was also in it to win. I thought we had an amazing filly.

Gary gave her a terrible ride. I've had jockeys from all eras watch the race and tell me he couldn't have put a horse in more trouble if you tried: rushed, checked (held up), rushed, checked all through the race. It was very disappointing.

I always think about what would have happened if I had stayed with Jerry as her rider, a journeyman jock but someone who rode her to those two wins in Chicago. I live with that decision every day. If I could go back in time, Jerry would have ridden her. I am sorry on all accounts to Jerry, to Diana O., to Joe and Dom.

I know there's some racetrack truisms, such as you never name a horse after a person and you should always sell if you are offered the chance because you never know what can happen if you turn down the offer. My attitude was if something was going to happen after not selling the horse, it's going to happen. Do I look back and say, "Yeah, I should have taken the $250,000"? It's easy to say that now. We had her insured for $50,000, but big deal. There was no doubt in my mind she was a top two-year-old filly—I'm talking a horse that was capable of winning a Breeders' Cup major stakes—and it was just bad luck. Before there were great fillies such as Zenyatta and Rachel Alexandra; Diana O. was on that level. That I know 100 percent.

Should we have stayed in Chicago and run in a race other than a stakes, or lay her up for the season and get her ready for her three-year-old season? I guess so, but it's all hindsight now.

A few hours after the Diana O. tragedy, I arrived at the arena and all my teammates wanted to know how Diana O. did. I told them and it was not a good scene inside that dressing room. The guys knew I was torn apart. We lost 7–6 in overtime and, somehow, despite being pissed off, I had two goals and three assists in the game. I scored the game's opening goal at 3:51 of the first period and retrieved the puck for sentimental reasons and wrote DIANA O. on tape wrapped around the puck as a tribute to her.

I went home after the game and was so distraught, just sick to my stomach. Joe and Dom were also upset. Joe had flown in for the race from Chicago and planned to fly back, but decided to drive back and go home with Dom, who had driven to the race. Before getting into the car they noticed the back right tire was flat. Diana O. had broken her right hind leg, so when you think about the flat tire being the back right, it's pretty eerie. A long ride home, for sure.

Darren Dunn, my friend from Assiniboia Downs, recalls me showing him a recording of the race and how my eyes welled up and I had to look away. He says it was an example of how I was a tough and fit NHL player and yet I was emotionally brought to my knees by a young horse that I had become attached to, combined with never knowing how good she might have been.

After Diana O., it took me five years to get back into the game at all levels—owning horses, betting horses, watching races. It was really hard. Did I start going back to the races? Yeah. Did I own anything? No. Was my heart in it? No. You feel like you've done everything right and something like that happens. Should we have scratched the filly out of the race because of the weather conditions? Because the filly had been named after Diana also made it hard.

Thoroughbreds are bred to race, but that was rough. You don't get many opportunities, especially with a horse like that. We got her at a bargain price and she won her first two races easily and then it all changed.

* * *

Similar to what we did in Toronto, we lived in Winnipeg in the off-season except for a four-week period during which we went back home. We had become entrenched in the community. Life was pretty good at this point and I was really looking forward to my first full season in Winnipeg.

DIANA OLCZYK
Eddie's wife

One of the best things that ever happened to us was being traded to Winnipeg. We loved Winnipeg. The people were phenomenal. The team was close-knit. The guys were gone for two to three weeks at a time and the wives would all rally together and became really close. A lot of us had small children, so we'd hang out at Chuck E. Cheese.

Something funny happened in the preseason. My horse Mr. Bow Tie was running at Arlington, but they had no simulcast racing or online wagering in Winnipeg at Assiniboia Downs. I found an off-track betting shop at a Best Western Motel in Grand Forks, North Dakota. We had the horse entered in a $12,000 claiming running about a mile on the turf. He could win for a $25,000 tag on the grass, but couldn't win for a $5,000 tag on the dirt. We had tried to get him on the grass for a higher tag a couple of times, but the races didn't fill with enough starters.

The day that he was running, the Jets were scheduled to play a preseason game out of town. I knew this a few days before. I had already played a couple of preseason games, so I asked John if I could be excused from the game. I told him I'd play in the next preseason game, and that our horse had a really good shot to win and that I'd bet a few bucks for him. He told me it was no problem.

We had an early practice that day before the game on race day and I showed up for practice to look at the line combinations. I noticed I was scheduled to play. I went to see John right away and told him I couldn't play because I was driving to Grand Forks. He said he forgot and made a change so I wouldn't have to play. I got in my car and drove the three hours from Winnipeg.

I had about $1,500 U.S. on me, including my own cash and some from my teammates, and had to wait for the 10th and final race on the card. I bet Mr. Bow Tie, who went postward at more than 9-1 odds, to win, place, and in exactas. He won by a neck with jockey Jerry La Sala and paid $20.40 to win (on a $2 investment), $8.40 to place, and combined for a $130.40 exacta for $2. They had to write me an IOU for about $20,000 because they only had about $7,800 in the till. It was an off-track betting shop in a hotel. What a country! I paid John and some of the other guys on the team. Somebody else was going to Grand Forks later on and cashed in one of the IOUs for about $5,000. So, it was well worth the trip to Grand Forks and not having to dress for that preseason game. At least I scored off the ice that day. It felt really good, too.

DARREN DUNN
Assiniboia Downs CEO
Grand Forks is this beautiful little town and the teletheater was in a peanut bar. In walks a swashbuckling horseplayer guy and it's Eddie. First of all, the size of his wager probably shocked them, and when it hit there's no way they would have had that kind of money on hand.

Once the regular season started, I had eight goals and 12 assists in 25 games and was feeling pretty good. Then it happened again—I was traded. This time it was to the New York Rangers for tough wingers Tie Domi and Kris King, three days after Christmas. There were some rumors between Thanksgiving and Christmas I was on the block. If you are an NHL player and you really want to know what's going on, you talk to the trainers. I kept asking our trainer, Craig Heisinger, "Where am I going? Do you know everything? What nameplates do you have in your equipment truck?" I think he knew, but didn't let on that he did.

The day I was traded, I arrived for practice and John Paddock was waiting for me when I was going into the equipment room.

"I need to talk to you," he said.

I was thinking, please don't tell me I'm traded. I really love it here, the people, the team, you.

"I've got to inform you that we've traded you to the New York Rangers."

John Paddock was one of my best coaches. The type of guy John is, he came to my house once to tell me I was going to be a healthy scratch. He did not want to embarrass me at the rink. We were not playing well and I wasn't playing well, either. It was simply a matter of the team already having enough scoring depth up front. Teemu Selanne was there. It was his first season and he had nine goals in his first 10 games and was on his way to setting an NHL rookie record with 76 goals. Alexei Zhamnov was also in his rookie year and had seven assists in 10 games and was starting to score in December. Keith Tkachuk was in his first full season. We were on the cusp of doing something big and John said management felt we needed more toughness. In retrospect, filing for arbitration may have had something to do with the trade.

The timing was terrible. My mother-in-law, June Ann, had a stroke just before Christmas, so we were dealing with that over the holidays. I went home and told Diana and she broke down. She was obviously upset for a lot of different reasons, her mother's health being one of them. I told Rangers general manager Neil Smith about my situation and he allowed me to take a few days before I had to join the Rangers for their next game, which was New Year's Eve in Buffalo. I wanted to make sure Diana was okay.

I had a relationship with Rangers coach Roger Neilson because he was an assistant during my three years in Chicago. I had also done guest coaching at his hockey came in Peterborough, Ontario. When I joined the Rangers, I was told to see Roger.

The first thing he said to me was, "I just want to let you know when Neil came to me with this trade, I told him I didn't want to make it. I love Kris King."

I'm thinking, are you kidding me? I just left a place where I was playing and now I'm coming to a place where the coach didn't want to make the trade. I asked him if I was going to play and he said yes.

I made my debut on New Year's Eve on a line with Sergei Nemchinov and Adam Graves. I had been on a lot of teams and that was probably the first and only time I saw guys completely dog it in a game because they wanted to get the coach fired. I heard from a few guys prior to the game there was some tension around the team and coaches. The Rangers were captained by Mark Messier, who was not seeing eye to eye with Roger. We lost 11–6. The guys either knew Roger was about to get fired or felt they had to get embarrassed big time and then the coach would be fired. I was thinking, what the hell have I gotten myself into?

After we lost our next game, 5–2 against Pittsburgh two days later, Neil fired Roger and transferred him into a scouting role. He was replaced by Ron Smith, the head coach of the Rangers' American Hockey League farm team in Binghamton. The team had a record of 19–17–4 at the time. Smith finished with a record of 15–22–7 in 44 games and we missed the playoffs.

It was one of those things where if you are playing and having success and your family is happy, it doesn't matter how much money you are making. That's the best-case scenario. I finished with 13 goals and 16 assists in 46 games for the Rangers and overall scored 21 goals with 28 assists.

I was invited by Team USA general manager Brian Burke to play and be the captain for the team in the 1993 World Championships. What a great honor and I thank Burkie for doing that. Tim Taylor was the head coach and our team included Tony Amonte, Derian Hatcher, Mike

Modano, Mike Richter, and Doug Weight, among others. Even though we didn't qualify for the playoffs it was still a great experience. Whenever Team USA invited me to represent my country, I accepted all but one time, and that was only because I was recovering from a back injury. I encourage every American-born hockey player who is asked to play for their country in any world competition to do it. Obviously certain situations arise, but if you can, just go play.

Ronnie Salcer and I went to arbitration in the off-season and because of the Collective Bargaining Agreement between the owners and the players, I wasn't able to use the statistics from the year that just passed. The year I just played did not exist in this arbitration. Technically, I had just played a season without a contract. Jets GM Mike Smith, who traded me, and Rangers GM Neil Smith, who acquired me, were going to present arguments. So, Mike Smith is negotiating a contract for another team because I am a New York Ranger. The GM of one team is representing another team? Yep. That's pretty messed up. Not a lot of people know this story and I'm sure they're wondering how a player could play with no contract and then go to arbitration for a year that didn't even exist. It's absolutely crazy.

Ronnie had prepared me ahead of time what would unfold and warned that it could get ugly, but he had a game plan. My friend Joe was at the hearing, too. I had a great team representing me. Mike Smith started ripping me and I wasn't even a Jets player anymore. It was incredible. A lot of the stuff that was said in the hearing was personal. It's business, I get it. There were times when I was ready to lose it—I think one time I blurted out "That's a lie"—but Ronnie kept me in check to make sure I kept my cool. It's easier to be bad-mouthed by someone who *is* your boss than someone who *was* your boss.

The Jets offered me something like $375,000, about a $25,000 increase on my salary. Neil Smith tried to come to terms with Ronnie, offering more than the Jets, but Ronnie wouldn't budge because I was a consistent 30-goal scorer.

After Mike Smith talked, carving me up for some 25 minutes, Ronnie began his presentation. It only lasted five minutes—and we had the ace! He had a big easel with a cover sheet over it and he lifted it up and said over the course of the last five seasons in the NHL, there had only been seven players who scored 30 or more goals in each. He had seven sheets with a name on each and began to pull the sheets back one at a time with each name: Wayne Gretzky, Pat LaFontaine, Luc Robitaille, Steve Yzerman, Mike Gartner, Brett Hull, and one more player. And he lifts the final page and it's my name. Yep, Eddie Olczyk. Pretty good company I might say; those guys are all Hall of Famers. That list still looks great 30 years later.

It had all unfolded exactly the way Ronnie told me before the meeting and Mike Smith was dumbfounded. Those other players were making at least $1 million. Some guys were making $3 million. The arbiter ruled I would get a two-year deal worth $850,000 a season. So, the Rangers had to cut me a check for $500,000 to pay back the money owed to me from the prior season.

After all that, I was feeling pretty good about my salary.

But I could never have imagined what would happen next in New York.

CHAPTER 9

No More 1940

WHEN I LOOK BACK ON MY CAREER, I can say the beginning of the end happened in New York in the 1993–94 season, the year I was a member of the Rangers team that won the Stanley Cup. I celebrated a dream that every player has from the time they begin to play the game and pursue it professionally. Individually, however, it proved to be a trying experience and tested my resolve and love of the game.

Basically, it was all because of Mike Keenan.

On April 17, 1993, the Rangers announced the hiring of Keenan as their new coach. He had coached previously in Philadelphia and Chicago, making it to the Stanley Cup Final three times. He had been out of hockey for a year and there had been rumors that the Rangers were going to hire him. In his career, he had developed a reputation for being tough on players.

In training camp, Keenan had a full team meeting at the practice facility in Rye Playland in Rye, New York. A TV with a VCR was brought out and he showed video of all the championship parades New York sports teams had enjoyed in the past. The Rangers had last won the Stanley Cup in 1940. Journey's famed song, "Don't Stop Believin'," was playing in the background, and collectively it was a great video with great music. Extremely well played.

Keenan basically said, "You win at this and you'll walk together for the rest of our lives." When the video ended, everybody was all jacked up and then Keenan started walking around the room and addressing the players individually.

He said to Mark Messier, "You're our captain and you're going to score the game-winning goal in Game 7 of the Stanley Cup and you're going to be the first one from the Rangers to touch the Cup in 54 years."

Then he looked at Mike Richter and said, "You're going to stop every puck that comes your way."

He turned to Adam Graves and said, "You're going to score 50 goals."

He told Brian Leetch, "You're going to be the best defenseman in the NHL."

He looked at Joey Kocur and said, "You're going to beat the crap out of anybody who touches Mark Messier."

Everybody laughed and then he looked at me and said, "Eddie Olczyk"—and then there was a long pause. It seemed like five minutes, but it was only five seconds.

And then he said, "You may not play all season long, but you're going to have a role on this team."

Right away, I knew I was in trouble: He had his mind made up about me. I was going to be a Black Ace, the hockey term used for players who are extras. I knew that no matter what I did, I wasn't going to get to play on a regular basis. But I learned in my career that when you are part of a team, there's two things you've got to do: you've got to accept your role, and you've got execute it.

Was I upset? Absolutely. But I never let my teammates hear it. I wanted to play but that opportunity wasn't going to be there, so I decided to just work hard and keep my mouth shut. My role that year was to make the guys laugh and lead the guys in the stretching before the practices. I started saying "Heave-ho," meaning let's pull together, as our mantra.

MIKE HARTMAN
Eddie's teammate

He started stretching the guys out and I made a joke once to him because he was kind of miserable. I said, "Eddie, how many personal trainers out there make $850,000 a year to stretch people in the morning?" He didn't really think it was funny.

Forward Nick Kypreos, who was one of the Black Aces, says the stretches may have only lasted five or so minutes, but it's one of those quality moments for a team. He says what I did in the team stretch set the tone for the rest of the day and he always looked at me as being the leader of our little group.

NICK KYPREOS
Eddie's teammate

I don't know if another group of guys would have taken it as well as our group, and Eddie was the leader of that. There's two roads to take: the bad attitude one or the one that says, let's come to work and make the best of it. That's where Eddie was so good.

Whatever team I played on, I always appreciated every player regardless of how big or how small their role was. It was not easy to become one of those extra players. I had been a 30-goal scorer several times and now it was etched in stone that I wasn't going to play.

There were certain guys who Keenan liked and certain guys he didn't, and if you were one of the latter, he was going to make life miserable for you. Keenan was really hard on Leetch, Tony Amonte, Mike Gartner, and others. Early in the season, defenseman James Patrick, who had played nine full seasons for New York, and center Darren Turcotte, who had played more than four seasons, were traded to Hartford for Kypreos, fellow forward Steve Larmer, defenseman Barry Richter, and a draft pick. Keenan wanted Larmer, whom he coached in Chicago, for his scoring. Chicago traded Larmer to Hartford and the Whalers then traded him to New York. It all happened the same day.

I began the season as a healthy scratch and after about five or six games I went to see Keenan in his office to find out if there was anything I could do to get some minutes. He was there with his assistants, Dick Todd and Colin Campbell, and had his feet up on his desk. I spilled my guts. It was very emotional, and while I told him this he was looking out into the sound, because the practice facility is right by the water. I was dressed in a suit and after I'd been talking for about five minutes, he pulled his feet off the desk, stood up, leaned over, and said, "You done?"

I said, "Yes."

He leaned over and looked at my shoes, which were black with some striping across the front of them.

"Your shoes," he said. "Is that alligator on the top of them?"

"I have no idea," I replied.

"Okay, see you later, alligator," he said.

I just walked out of there shaking my head and thinking, what an a-hole. He did not hear one word I said.

It was typical Keenan.

***

GLENN HEALY
Eddie's teammate

We each had roles and I think Eddie could have given Christmas mass at the Vatican and Mike still wouldn't have cared. He already had a pre-disposed idea of what Eddie's role was going to be, if he even had one, and I would argue he didn't have one. No matter what Eddie had done it wouldn't have mattered, even though his career was spectacular up to that point.

We had a record of four wins and three losses in the first seven games, and in the eighth game Keenan was incensed. We were playing the expansion Mighty Ducks of Anaheim, which had a record of 1–2–2 after five games. During the game, he was so angry he essentially stopped coaching and the guys on the bench had to change the lines. I dressed for this game and remember him saying during the second period, "Excuse me, excuse me, you guys don't need me, coach yourselves." It was his way of saying, you guys think you are so good, you can coach yourselves. I immediately thought, great, I will play a regular shift finally. We lost 4–2.

I was a healthy scratch for all but four of the team's first 13 games, then played in six consecutive games. Starting with the 12th game of the season, we started to really come together, winning seven in a row en route to a franchise record at that time with 52 wins and 112 points. But Keenan was always on edge.

I remember one game against Philly, in which I was a healthy scratch. We won but Keenan wasn't happy. Aside from three bad minutes, we played really well. The guys were having a good time on the bus back to New York and we popped in the movie *Stripes*. Keenan told Dick Todd to get up and shut the movie off. Todd stood up and stopped the movie and I started the booing and everybody on the bus started to boo as well. Keenan wanted to see how the team would react by stopping the movie. I was sitting in the middle of the bus and knew my role, so I started a chant of "Stripes, Stripes, Stripes." Then the whole team started to chant, "Stripes, Stripes, Stripes." We did it for about 15 seconds and it was getting louder and louder and louder. You could see Keenan throwing his hands up in the air in frustration and then he told Dick to put the movie back on. Todd stood up and the guys started cheering. I figured I should tweak it one more time and started singing "For He's a Jolly Good Fellow." The guys absolutely roared. Our bus driver, Ricky, later told us he looked at Keenan when we were singing and he had a huge grin on his face. Ricky said it was priceless. Again, this was Keenan playing mind games to see how the team would react. Did he have to tell Dick Todd to shut the movie off? No. But that's what we dealt with.

Greg Gilbert, who was a forward on the team, says the smiles and laughter that I brought to the dressing room every day were hilarious. I was just trying to keep the guys loose.

Beginning in our 22nd game of the season, I started to play regularly and score some points. There was one game, our 44th of the season, in Chicago that sticks out in my mind. It was Steve Larmer's first game back facing his former team. I should note Steve Larmer is a great human and great teammate who should be in the Hockey Hall of Fame, without question. He was so smooth with the puck. If you were in trouble and had the puck, just get it to Larms. Anyway, I was very talkative on the bench, always trying to help guys on the ice in all situations, being the eyes and ears for the guys, yelling, "Heads up" and "Icing," letting everybody know what was going on. It was the second period and I'm on the bench and I see an icing play develop and I start yelling "Icing" as loud as I can. All of a sudden, I see the linesman put his arm down and wave it off. So now I'm yelling, with a touch of panic in my voice, "No icing."

And then, bam, the puck ends up on the stick of Hawks forward Dirk Graham and he scores on Mike Richter. We were winning 3–1, but Keenan was pissed. I could feel him walking toward me calling me stupid a couple of times and telling me the goal was my fault because I yelled from the bench. That got my goat. I had a teacher call me stupid once and it really bothered me. I don't like that word at all.

Keenan told me to not to say another word.

The next time the puck was shot down the ice I yelled "Icing" twice as loud. Screw him. I wasn't going to stop being myself and was going to do what I could to help the team. We won the game 5–1 and Larms scored on a penalty shot on Eddie Belfour.

Keenan enjoyed seeing how people reacted when he was behind the bench or in public. I had never played for a coach like that before. He was pretty rough and you had to have thick skin.

We had such a great group of guys who would pick up your spirits if Keenan ever embarrassed you. Some guys he picked on, some guys he genuinely didn't like, and some guys he knew could take it. The only guy he never went after was Mess.

Even when I started playing regularly, I never felt it would last. I knew I was on fragile ground with Keenan. It was almost like I was just killing time. He'd get you so wound up, you'd start doing stuff that was outside your character.

Four games after Chicago, we were in Anaheim and he got in my ear saying, "When are you going to do something around here?" I said, "When you start playing me." I hadn't played in seven or eight minutes and he was playing mind games. Like an idiot, on my next shift we iced the puck and I tried to outrace the defenseman to negate the icing. Keenan got me so wound up I decided to dive for the puck headfirst 10 feet from the boards. I negated the icing, but went crashing into the boards. My right hand hit the wall first and shattered my thumb. When I got back to the bench my thumb was sitting south and I pulled it out of the glove and it was coming out of my wrist. It was some serious pain.

Our head trainer, Dave Smith, came over to help me out. He suggested we have the Ducks' doctor check me out. I was more shocked than anything else. As I was getting up to go to the dressing room, Keenan said, "Where the hell are you going?" I said my thumb was messed up and he said, "You sit here, we need some moral support." So, like an 'idiot, I did. I sat there for probably eight minutes opening the door at the end of the bench with my left hand while holding up my throbbing right hand above my shoulder. I finally went into the dressing room at the end of the period. I had played 36 games at that point and had three goals and five assists. Now I was sidelined indefinitely after undergoing surgery.

At the March deadline, general manager Neil Smith made a bunch of trades, very good ones I might add, acquiring talented players who were also great human beings. These were players Keenan wanted: Craig MacTavish from Edmonton, Glenn Anderson from Toronto, and Stephane Matteau and Brian Noonan from Chicago. Todd Marchant, Mike Gartner, and Tony Amonte were traded away. I didn't know how it was all going to shake out for me, but when I saw the experienced guys they brought in, the window to play probably was slammed shut unless a couple of guys got hurt. It really didn't matter what I did, I wasn't going to play and I had to figure out how to help this team. I was one of the Black Aces again and had to do whatever I could to help the team and wait for my chance.

Ray Ferraro, who played with the New York Islanders at the time and later became my teammate and linemate in Los Angeles, says it seemed at that time like our team was getting better and better, and when they made the moves at the deadline guys like me kind of got left on the outside.

It's often said a person shows his true colors when things don't go their way. That was my attitude all along and it's something I've tried to teach my kids.

The final regular season game ended in a 2–2 tie with Philadelphia. We finished first overall in the league with 52 wins, 24 losses, and eight ties.

I was voted the Players' Player by the team at a dinner before the playoffs started. It was an annual team award and I was so honored to be recognized by my teammates, my peers. That was the individual highlight of my professional life, earning the respect of some amazing hockey players and people who appreciated my role and what I did. I couldn't be prouder of that. I had very little impact on the ice, but obviously they thought I was important and recognized me for that.

* * *

We faced the New York Islanders in the first round and it was my chance to truly experience the rivalry the Rangers had with them. The Islanders won four Cups in the 1980s and their fan base is off the charts. They liked to taunt the Rangers and their playoff drought with a "1940" chant, the last time our franchise had won the Cup. Ferraro recalls thinking his Islanders team had no chance against our lineup just based on the talented players who were sitting out.

I didn't play in the series, but I was there watching and it was really intense. We beat the Islanders 5–4 in early March, the first time a Rangers team had defeated them in their arena in almost five years. The intensity was like a playoff game. Now it was the playoffs, but we beat them four straight, scoring 22 goals and only giving up three. Mike Richter recorded shutouts in the first two games.

We then played Washington and won the first three games before losing our first game of the playoffs. But we rebounded to win the next game and the series. We faced New Jersey in the conference final and we were pretty confident because we won all six games against them in the regular season. But like I said before, the playoffs are a totally different animal and those were the Devils, another archrival just 50 miles from New York City.

We knew it was going to be a long series against New Jersey and the Devils won the first game 4–3 with Stephane Richer scoring the game-winner in double overtime. They gained a lot of traction and we knew it was going to take everything we had to stop that momentum. The silver lining was that we only played four games against the Islanders and five against the Capitals, so we had a lot left in the tank if it was going to be a seven-game series.

We won the second game 4–0 and the third game 3–2 in overtime on a goal by Stephane Matteau. The Devils came back and won Game 4, which became a pivotal moment in the season and our run for the Cup.

After the Devils took a 2–0 lead in the first period, Keenan replaced Richter with Glenn Healy. He later benched Brian Leetch, and according to the guys and what I saw from the pressbox, Keenan stopped coaching, something he'd done on a few occasions earlier in the season. He didn't talk to anybody in his typically arrogant way. That's what he would do when things weren't going well.

I was a healthy scratch, and just watching you could just see what was going on and wondering why Leetch wasn't playing. It was really embarrassing. It was only 2–0; big deal. With all the talent we had, we only needed one goal to get back in it. Keenan quit coaching in the middle of a playoff series. He made a comment to the media that Leetch had an undisclosed injury, but Leetch said he didn't. It was a pretty tenuous situation.

In the documentary *Road to Victory: The 1994 New York Rangers Story*, Keenan said the controversial moves he's made in his career were instinctual. He said there were some moves made because of injuries and some to get the team more motivated and prepared for what was to come. He summed it up by saying, "That's coaching."

Leetch offered his own thoughts in the documentary and said Keenan made a bad decision. He admitted he'd never played a perfect game in his career and that it's certainly a coach's job to send messages, but that we were beyond that at this point in the playoffs.

I was completely shocked that Keenan would do that in a game of that magnitude. After Game 4 we were all in the dressing room after the loss and the room was super quiet. Keenan said a few things and then asked if anyone had anything to say. Even though I hadn't played, I thought in my role as a leader I should say something.

"Look, it's 2–2 in the series," I said. "It's a best of three, we're going home and we're going to win at home and have a 3–2 lead in the series and we're going to come back here again for Game 6 and win it and go to the Stanley Cup Final. We've got to be in this thing together. Let's stick together."

The reference to sticking together was a direct shot at the coach after the selfish b.s. antics he pulled. He got real defensive and got right into my face.

"What are you saying, Eddie? Are you saying I'm not loyal?"

He wanted me to call him out for what he did or how he coached in that game. Without saying he quit on everybody, I just said, "We've all got to stick together."

I know what I wanted to say to him, but that wasn't the time. The guys certainly knew what I was saying and I think he got the message that what he did was uncalled for. He could have easily torn the team apart and missed an opportunity to win a Stanley Cup.

The next day there was an optional skate and stretch. Mess went in to talk to Keenan and pretty much said what he did was b.s. and couldn't happen again. He told Keenan that he couldn't be quitting in a game and benching Leetch down by only two goals.

Mess came in late during the stretch and said, "Guys, what happened last night will never happen again." And that was it and we started stretching again.

We lost Game 5 at home and were now one defeat from elimination. Brian Noonan was hurt and I was standing at the stick rack the morning of Game 6, getting ready to go on the ice for the morning skate, when Keenan came over to me. Out of the blue he asked, "What's your best goal-scoring year in the NHL?"

I said, "I scored 42 goals with the Leafs."

He was in disbelief. Sarcastically, he asked, "You scored 42 goals one year in the NHL?"

"Yeah, I scored 30-plus goals for five years until I came here."

"You're playing tonight, I trust you. The guys trust you. You're in."

"Wow, I wish I would have got you a media guide before the season started and maybe I might have played a little bit more if you realized how many goals I scored."

He kind of laughed and walked away.

He knew he was going to play me all along. It was just another mind game.

The media spoke to Mark and he was asked by one of the reporters what had to happen for the team to win Game 6. Mark said, "We're going to go in there and win Game 6. We've done that all year. We've won all the games we've had to win. I know we're going to go in and win Game 6 and bring it back [home] for Game 7. We have enough talent and experience to turn the tide."

Many of the guys had no idea what had happened until they read the newspaper the next day. The *New York Post* ran a huge headline: "'We'll Win Tonight': Captain Courageous' Bold Prediction." In 2012, *Post* writer Mark Everson wrote a retrospective story that explained the headline of Mess' prediction produced one of the paper's most memorable pages for the sports section.

"That moment passed almost unnoticed as he handled more intelligent questions with more in-depth answers, but that quiet certainty, and his hat-trick fulfillment of it the next night, created a legend that still lives large in Rangers lore and haunts the Devils," Everson wrote in the story.

It was a guarantee that would be remembered the same way Joe Namath's was before the New York Jets beat the Baltimore Colts in Super Bowl III. Of course, Broadway Joe delivered on his promise.

Before the game in the dressing room, it was dead quiet. Kevin Lowe broke the silence when he said, "Well, Mess, I guess we've got to win this one."

Many of the guys had won Cups before with Edmonton, and Mess predicting we would win kind of broke the tension. It was pretty cool, it really was. We just wanted to give ourselves a chance to get back home. That's all we wanted to do.

Richter put on one of the greatest goaltending performances that I have ever seen playing or working a playoff game. The Devils led 2–0 after the first period, but it should have been 4–0. Richter was awesome. Alex Kovalev scored late in the second period to make it 2–1 and that gave us the hope and belief we could come back. And then Mess delivered on his promise. He scored on a backhand at 2:48 of the third to tie the game, then scored the go-ahead goal at 12:12 on a rebound. The Devils pulled Martin Brodeur with less than two minutes to go. Messier took the faceoff to the right side of Richter and won the draw. The puck came around to the other side and he got possession of it just below the faceoff circle, and fired it into the open net with 1:45 left on the clock. Mess recorded a natural hat trick on his 14th career shorthanded goal in the playoffs, which set a record. We all gathered around him when he returned to the bench.

Game 6 would go down as not only a great win for our team, but one of the most memorable games in the history of the National Hockey League and all of sports. To be a part of that game, which ended up becoming the only one I played in that playoffs, was exhilarating. That's why you play. It was just crazy. I didn't know whether I would play again in the series because I didn't know what was going to happen with Brian Noonan. Maybe Keenan would stick with a winning lineup.

Game 7 was also historic. Brian Leetch opened the scoring at 9:31 of the second period with an amazing goal, doing a 360-degree spin around Bill Guerin and beating Brodeur between the legs. The Devils tied it up with 7.7 seconds to go in the third on a goal by Valeri Zelepukin.

Before the OT started, Stephane Matteau was one of the last dressed players to leave the dressing room. Some of the extra guys were around as intermission ended and I saw Matty on the way out. In broken English, he said, "Eddie, give me some luck." I grabbed his stick and put my lips on the blade, gave it a big kiss, and said, "Go get 'em, Matty."

At 4:24 of the second overtime period, Matty curled around the Devils' net to try a wraparound goal from the side of the crease and the puck banked off New Jersey defenseman Slava Fetisov and went by Brodeur on the blocker side.

Howie Rose, the Rangers radio play-by-play man, shouted: "Matteau, Matteau, Matteau! Stephane Matteau! And the Rangers have one more hill to climb, baby, but it's Mount Vancouver! The Rangers are headed to the Final!"

Rangers fans remember that as one of the greatest calls in all of sports broadcasting history.

* * *

Four days later we opened the Stanley Cup Final against the Vancouver Canucks. Vancouver finished second in the Pacific Division with 85 points, winning 41, losing 40, and tying three. They were coached by Pat Quinn and captained by Trevor Linden. Their team included Pavel Bure—the Russian Rocket—who led the league in goals. The Canucks had beaten the Calgary Flames, St. Louis Blues, and Toronto Maple Leafs to advance to the Final. Their series against Calgary went the full seven games, with the last three ending in OT and the final game in double OT with Bure netting the winner. The Canucks followed that up by defeating St. Louis and Toronto in five games apiece. They had a week in between their conference final and the start of the Stanley Cup Final. We had beaten them twice that season, 6–3 and 5–2.

There's no better feeling than being four wins away from winning the Cup. That's why you play. Regardless of how many games you play, there's nothing like playing in the Final. It's the pinnacle of the game. You know when you're practicing you're trying to win the hardest trophy to win in all of sports.

We were the best team all year long and there was all this talk of the Rangers not having won the Cup since 1940. I didn't know if my number would be called like it was in Game 6 of the New Jersey series. I don't want to say it's harder not playing, but it's not exactly comfortable. You don't have a hand in the result and you're pulling for the guys. You know what's going on and you're living and dying with every shift.

We lost the opening game of the series 3–2 in overtime. Canucks goalie Kirk McLean had the game of his life. We won the second game 3–1 to tie up the series and were headed to Vancouver.

We were scheduled to leave for Vancouver from Newark the day before Game 3. As we pulled away from the gate and taxied to the runway, our director of team services, Matty Loughran, came up to me on the plane and said Keenan wanted to see me. I was wondering what was going on. Was he going to trade me somehow? I walked to the front of the plane and he said, "Your wife is having some complications with the pregnancy, do you want to get off the flight?"

What a question. What do you think? Diana was really early into her pregnancy with Alexandra during that time, so I was worried. I had no idea what the complications were.

"What are you going to do?" Keenan asked.

"What do you mean what am I going to do?" I said. "I'm getting off this airplane and I'm going to see my wife."

Diana had contacted the team, and the Rangers contacted the charter service to get word to the plane.

A New Jersey state trooper came to the side of the airplane, the door opened, and I got out. The team set up a car to take me home. Diana had some intermittent bleeding going on and they didn't know exactly what it was. I rushed home and we went to the doctor and everything seemed to be fine. I got on a plane later that night.

We won both games in Vancouver, 5–1 and 4–2, to go home leading the series 3–1. In Game 4, with the Canucks leading 2–1 in the second period, Mike Richter stopped Bure on a penalty shot, a signature save of the playoffs, sticking out his right leg. Sergei Zubov scored a power-play goal for us later in the period to tie the game 2–2 and we scored two more goals in the third to win 4–2.

We had a chance to win the Cup at home in Game 5 and tickets were going for about $10,000 each. It was crazy. The city was up for grabs—parade routes in place, parties planned by everyone.

There was no scoring in the first period and then we fell behind 3–0 with about 17 minutes to go. We somehow got back even on goals by Doug Lidster, Steve Larmer, and Mark Messier and then Vancouver scored three to win the game. Now we had to fly all the way back across the country.

We probably played our worst game of the year and lost the next game 4–1. The saving grace for us was that there were two days in between Games 6 and 7, instead of one. That really helped us out. In fairness to Vancouver, they had a lot of flying for their games leading up to the Final. We had to bus to Long Island, fly to Washington, bus to New Jersey, and then fly to Vancouver. They got the short straw with all the travel.

Now all of a sudden it was like, maybe we're not going to win the Cup. Everybody was talking about the curse of 1940 and that we were going to blow it. But that extra day really helped out—rest matters physically and mentally—and we relied on our experience.

We took a 2–0 lead after the first period on goals by Brian Leetch and Adam Graves. Vancouver scored a shorthanded goal five minutes into the second period, but we went ahead 3–1 about eight minutes later on a power-play goal by Mark Messier with some help from a nearby Noonan. Vancouver scored a power-play goal about five minutes into the third, but Mike Richter made some amazing saves and we didn't allow them another goal. We found a way to gut it out and win 3–2.

The crowd started chanting "1940," knowing the demons had finally been put to rest. One fan held up a sign that read Now I Can Die

IN PEACE. When Mess took the Cup from NHL commissioner Gary Bettman, he had the biggest grin on his face.

Brian Leetch became the first American-born player to win the Conn Smythe Trophy as the Most Valuable Player of the playoffs. There were many other players who helped in various ways. It was truly a group effort.

My role was very small, but I took pride in what I did.

If you look at the video of us winning the Cup, we're all yelling, "Heave-ho, heave-ho, heave-ho!"

Lifting the Cup was great. There's no better feeling as a player. That's why you put in all the hard work and the sweat and the sacrifice. I thought about all the people who helped me along the way to get to that point. When you see your teammates lifting the Cup and guys passing it to you, it's like time stands still. You just think about a lot of things. You think you know what it takes to win until you actually do it and then you stand there and think to yourself, man, this is way harder than I ever thought.

Was the Cup heavy? Oh, yeah. You better have a good grip on it.

In the dressing room, Alex Kovalev held up the Cup and said, "No more 1940."

It was a heck of a celebration in the locker room. The champagne was flowing. It was only the second time in my life that I drank alcohol on purpose.

This was the moment we had all dreamed of when we started playing hockey and now it had happened. We walked out of the Garden at 5:00 in the morning and there were fans on the street waiting to see us.

We went on a bender in New York immediately after winning. We'd get into a limo with the Cup and pull it out and put it on the hood of the car. We stopped traffic and people jumped out of their cars just to touch it. Everywhere we went, it was the people's trophy, New York's trophy. Whether it was in restaurants or bars, we wanted to share it with everybody. The Cup was a magnet and people wanted to touch it and thank us. It was awesome.

The parade was planned for three days later on June 17. That morning, Diana, Eddie, Tommy, and I got into a car and drove down to Madison Square Garden. We took a bus and then stepped onto a float. We were at the Canyon of Champions and Wall Street and I can't tell you if there were a million or 2 million people lining the parade route. In a video that is available online of the parade, broadcaster Marv Albert said 1.5 million people lined the streets and that we were the toast of the town. It was a mass of humanity and ticker tape was flying everywhere. It was the bomb, nothing better. It was a really hot day and we all had on our jerseys, but we were feeling great. On the parade route, I was on a float with Esa Tikkanen and Dougie Lidster and their families and we were waving and whooping it up and having a good time.

Diana, Eddie, and Tommy were with me on the float, and Eddie pulled on my shorts and said, "Dad, I just want to say thanks for inviting all these people to my birthday party." June 17 was his birthday and he thought all those people were there for him.

I said, "Eddie, you're welcome, but this will be the biggest birthday party you will ever have." That I'll never forget.

We got to City Hall, and we all went up on a stage and Mayor Rudy Giuliani was there. We got keys to the city, some members of the team spoke, and fans were chanting "Four more years!" at Keenan. Al Trautwig of MSG Network was there introducing everybody, and when I was introduced—and for the record I was not on the speakers' list, but I knew my role—I walked right to the podium and said, "One is unbelievable, there's only one thing better and that's two—heave-ho, two in a row, heave-ho, two in a row." It was kind of spur of the moment, but again, I knew my role.

While it was our win, it was also for the fans.

That day will be remembered for other reasons: O.J. Simpson went on his Bronco journey down a California highway and the New York

Knicks were playing Game 5 of the National Basketball Association Finals against the Houston Rockets. Obviously, a lot of people didn't see the parade nationally because of what was happening with O.J. When I got home later that day, all anybody was talking about was the Bronco chase.

Every member of the team is allowed to take the Cup for 24 hours to do whatever they want. There's been some outrageous stories about players losing the Cup, eating ice cream and cereal out of it, or it ending up in a swimming pool.

Here's what I did: I went to the Meadowlands Racetrack on June 30 to have a private party with a few friends in a private room in the Pegasus dining area. The group included my buddies Dominic Porro and Scott Cooper and jockey Mike Luzzi. The harness racing meet was going on and star driver John Campbell came by. He's a huge New Jersey Devils fan and a season-ticket holder and he was very uncomfortable with the Stanley Cup being there. John took a picture but he wouldn't touch the Cup.

The next day, Dom and I drove from my home in a suburb of Rye to Belmont Park. The downtown area is maybe 400 yards long and the Rye Smoke Shop is right in the heart of the town. That's where I would pick up the *Daily Racing Form* whenever I would need it. I got to know a guy named Tony D'Oforio, whose folks owned the place, although he ran it. They were nice people and big Rangers fans—there were pictures of old Rangers players in there as well as my picture. I would describe the smoke shop, which closed in 2016 after more than 45 years in business, as probably the size of a walk-in closet, probably 40 feet long and 12 feet wide.

At that time, there wasn't anyone hired by the National Hockey League to look after the Cup—a position later called Keeper of the Cup—and no crate for carrying it. And if you're driving around with the Cup the way I did, you either strapped it into a seat belt or put it in the trunk of your car. That was just the reality of it. So, I put the Cup in the back of our Town & Country where we usually put the groceries. And if you picture driving into downtown Rye, you go up a little bit of a hill. Once you got to the top of the hill, you can see downtown Rye. As I'm driving the car, I look at Dominic and say, "Is there a parade going on downtown? Look at all the people."

There looked to be thousands of people. As we moved closer, I could see a fire engine with the ladders up and the sirens blaring. Then I began to wonder, how do they know I have the Stanley Cup in the car? There was an open spot for me to park my car right in front of the smoke shop.

Dom asked, "Who did you tell?"

I said, "I didn't tell anybody anything. All I said to Tony was, I might have a surprise for you next Friday. I didn't say I was bringing the Cup. I just said I might have a surprise."

When I got out of the car, the people erupted and Tony came flying out of the store and I said, "What's with all the people?"

"Eddie, I'm sorry, I only told one person," he said.

"I didn't say I was bringing the Cup."

"I kind of thought that that's what you were going to do."

"Jeez, I'm glad I didn't screw this up by not having the Cup."

There had to be 2,000 people on that corner. I opened the sliding door, picked up the Cup, and lifted it over my head as the whole crowd exploded. People were jumping up trying to touch it. I gave it to Tony and he took it into the shop and took a picture with it. We were there maybe 20 minutes and people passed the Cup around outside and took pictures with it.

It was so great to know you played a part in making so many people so happy. That memory will last a lifetime. That's something I will never forget. It was crazy. And I got my *Daily Racing Form*, as well.

I then brought the Cup to the Chase Bank and saw my banker. I also had to get some money to make some bets at the track.

Then we went to Belmont Park. The New York Racing Association allowed me to bring the Cup. NYRA also wanted to photograph the Cup

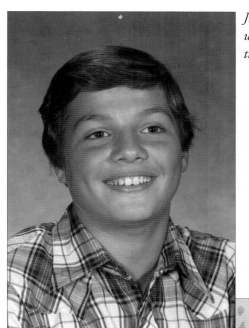

*Just a kid from Chicago
who lived and died with
the Blackhawks.*

*Visiting Santa with my
brothers, Ricky (left)
and Randy (right).*

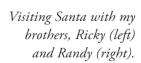

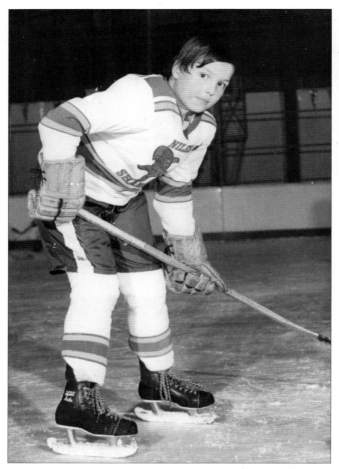

At the Ballard Sports Complex in Niles as a member of the Niles Sharks. Look at those gloves!

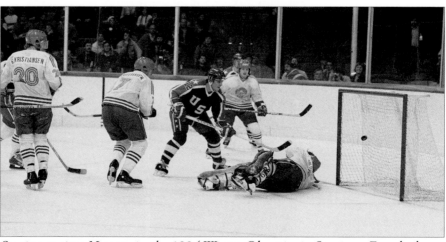

Scoring against Norway in the 1984 Winter Olympics in Sarajevo. Everybody told me I wouldn't make the team because I was too young, but I did. (AP Images)

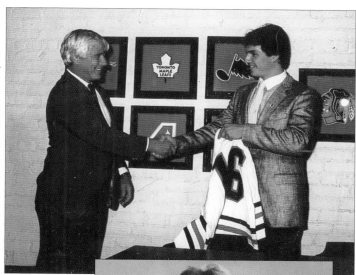

Shaking hands with Hawks GM Bob Pulford, who supported my attempt to make the '84 Olympic team and then made me the first American player drafted in the first round by his hometown team.

This is the autographed photo I got from Tom Lysiak after writing to him when I was 15 years old. Three years later, we were on a line together.

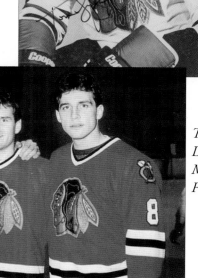

The Clydesdales Line: me, Troy Murray, and Curt Fraser.

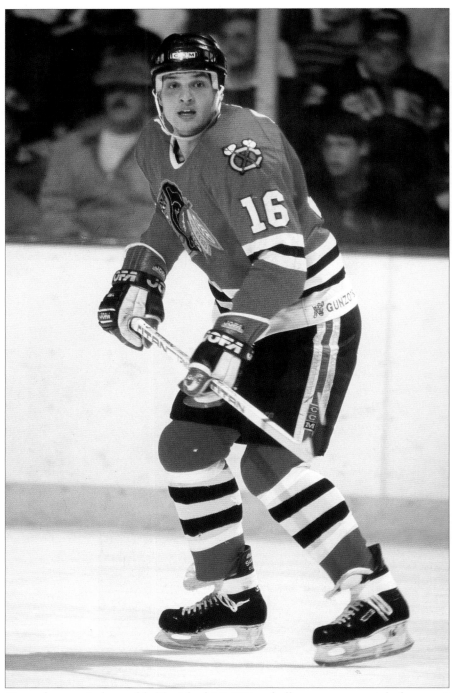

From day one I always felt like I had 36,000 eyeballs on me every night because I was a Chicago guy. I wanted to do so well for so many people, which was no easy task. (Getty Images)

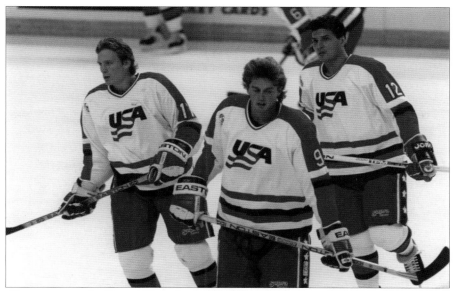

Skating again for Team USA, this time with Jeremy Roenick (left) and Mike Modano (center).

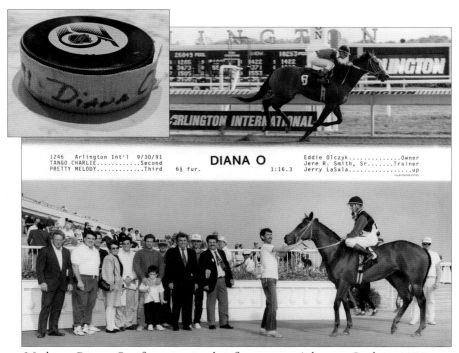

1246	Arlington Int'l	9/30/91	**DIANA O**		Eddie Olczyk	Owner
TANGO CHARLIE	Second				Jere R. Smith, Sr.	Trainer
PRETTY MELODY	Third	6½ fur.		1:16.3	Jerry LaSala	up

My horse Diana O. after winning her first race at Arlington Park in 1991. That's my best friend, Dominic Porro, on the far right wearing the sport coat and mustache. (Inset) The puck I saved in tribute to Diana O.

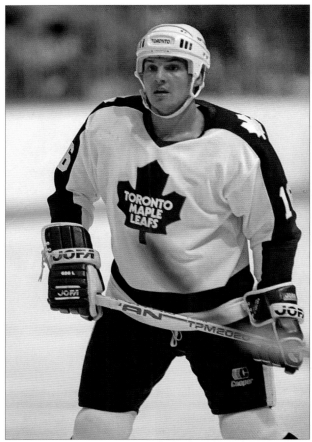

After three seasons in Chicago, being traded was the furthest thing from my mind. But I was sent to the Toronto Maple Leafs in 1987. At first I was crushed, but then I thought about playing for the Leafs and what a great opportunity it was.
(Getty Images)

After one of the worst playoff defeats in Leafs history, the fans threw all kinds of garbage onto the ice. After we won the next game, I told a reporter the fans should throw roses instead. They did. Our dog, Titan, didn't seem too impressed.

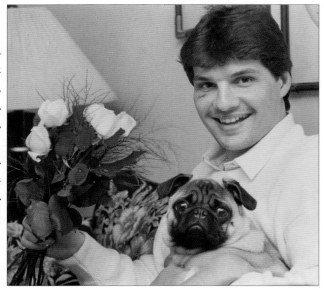

I didn't care for the way the Leafs handled my trade to the Jets, but we came to love our time in Winnipeg.

(Getty Images)

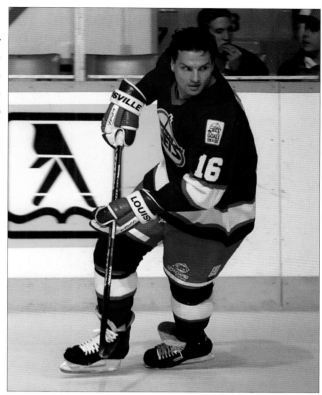

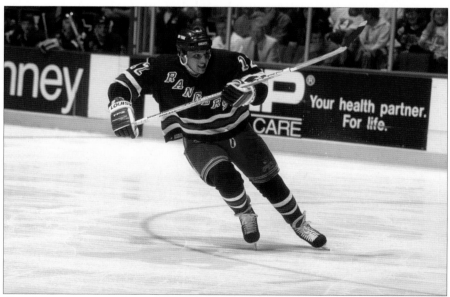

On the move again, this time to New York to play for the Rangers. Unfortunately, coach Mike Keenan had decided I wasn't going to play on a regular basis.
(Getty Images)

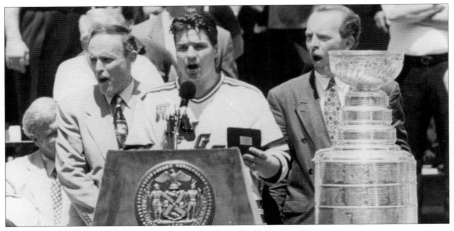

Despite not getting a lot of ice time, I did everything I could to help the team. It also didn't stop me from enjoying our Stanley Cup victory. At the championship rally with mayor Rudy Giuliani and Al Trautwig of MSG Network (top), with trainer Nick Zito and Kentucky Derby winner Go for Gin (middle), and meeting President Bill Clinton at the White House (bottom).

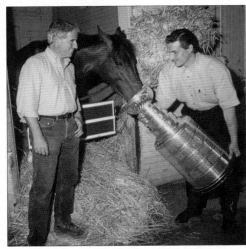

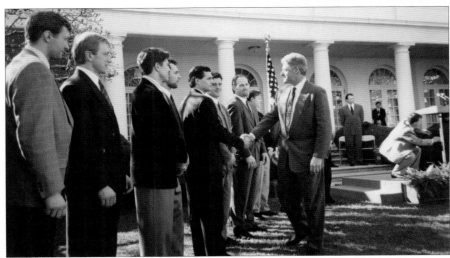

with 1994 Kentucky Derby winner Go for Gin, who was based in New York with trainer Nick Zito. NYRA thought it would be a great photo opportunity to show two champions of New York. I wanted to do it because going to the racetrack is what I loved to do away from hockey. I met Nick, whom I didn't know, at his barn, where he was with his son, Alex. Great people, a real thrill. We took a picture with Go for Gin in which his nose is in the Cup—we put some oats and hay in it prior to the photo—and it's one of my favorite photos.

Allen Gutterman, who was NYRA's vice president of marketing, worked it out so people could take a photo with the Cup by making a donation. We put the Cup at the finish line at the start of the day for the races and we let people take pictures for five hours. It felt like the line stretched from the winner's circle to Vancouver.

For as much as I think my career took a downward turn when I got to New York, I would not trade that year for anything because of the incredible teammates and friends and the whole experience. To bring a championship to New York—people had been waiting 54 years—that's as incredible as it gets.

I had already accepted that my name wasn't going to get engraved on the Cup because the rules said you had to play a minimum of 41 regular season games and/or play at least one game in the Final. But nobody was ever going to tell me that I wasn't a part of that team or my role wasn't important.

The players petitioned the NHL office to have my name and Mike Hartman's on the Cup. Adam Graves led the charge and he addressed it with Neil Smith, who relayed his thoughts to Mike Gartner. Neil thought Mike and I were a big part of the team all year and it was just not right that our names were not on the Cup. Gartner was the president of the NHL Players Association and had started out the season with the team until he was dealt by Neil to Toronto at the trade deadline. He spoke to NHL commissioner Gary Bettman during the lockout that delayed the start of the 1994–94 season and Mr. Bettman agreed to allow our names to be included. The names are usually inscribed on the Cup a few months after the season ends, so that is why if you look at the Cup, Mike and I have ours at the bottom of the list, after the trainers. But we may have set a precedent for players in similar situations.

Everybody had a role in winning the Stanley Cup. When we received our Stanley Cup rings, they had the words HEAVE-HO inscribed on the inside. Neil said when he designed the ring, he wanted to put 1940 with a slash through it to signify the end of the drought. He asked Mark if he wanted anything else to be on the ring and Mess said HEAVE-HO because that's what the players always said at practice.

We all pulled together and have a memory that will last forever.

* * *

The players knew there was a chance of a lockout before the 1994–95 NHL season because the owners wanted a salary cap and the NHL Players Association was against it. We played preseason games thinking there was going to be a regular season. I had a hat trick in one of those preseason games and felt good about my game. Then the lockout happened.

I was part of several work stoppages, strikes, or whatever you want to call them. It's not easy on anybody, but it's a big business and you'd like to think everybody wins. Owners, players, and fans don't want a work stoppage. As a player, you want to play, but it's just the nature of the beast.

I was really disappointed because of the training camp that I had and the preseason games. I was ready to bounce back after the past year of not playing and hoping to get back to where I was before I got traded to the Rangers.

But something really interesting happened to me. The Meadowlands Racetrack called and asked me if I wanted to work for them for the winter as part of the in-house broadcast of thoroughbred races. This is how I got my start in TV broadcasting.

Hal Handel, general manager of the New Jersey Sports and Exposition, which ran the Meadowlands Racetrack, contacted me about handicapping the live races in-house and on the recap show after the races. I knew Bruce Garland, the senior vice president of racing at the Meadowlands; Jimmy Gagliano, GM of administration and racing; and Chris McErlean, vice president of racing operations. They were all Rangers fans and they knew I was a horseplayer. I'd spent some time at the Meadowlands, whether it was the harness meet or the thoroughbred meet, and that's kind of how it all came together. I would be working three or four nights a week with Barbara Foster and Bob "Hollywood" Heyden, providing insights.

When they first asked me about it, my thought was, wow, they're going to pay me to go to the racetrack! I was going to come out to the track and handicap anyway, so it was a great fit. They were so gracious with the opportunity, but it was good publicity for them and it was a great experience for me. Who knew 20 years later I'd debut on NBC as part of its horse racing coverage, including the Triple Crown?

Michael Sheehan was our producer and it was interesting to see and experience the work that goes on behind the scenes. You're communicating with your co-host and the producer and director are talking to you through an inner earpiece called an IFB. I learned a lot in the three months I worked at the track. Was I a good handicapper? Sometimes. But some nights I couldn't pick a one-horse race correct. That's just horse racing. On one of the broadcasts I touted a 15-1 long shot that paid $30. There were times when I made good picks and people bet on them, and other times I'd be walking around and people told me I sucked. But that's all part of it. It's not easy to pick horses to win and there's pressure when you are asked to do it as part of a broadcast. All you can hope is that the same people who criticize you for your selections when they don't win have the same respect and courage to tell you that you've made a good pick when one of your choices wins. But it was fun and it was great to meet a lot of great people like trainers, jockeys, and racetrack officials. Considering there was no hockey going on, it ended up being a blessing in disguise for me.

At the start it was baby steps, for sure. Putting your opinion out for the world to see is great fun and pressure, just like getting the puck on your stick in an NHL game.

MICHAEL SHEEHAN
NBC producer

Eddie was terrific. Did I see something in him at the time that made me think he had a future as a broadcaster? Yeah. Did I think he would excel to become the top analyst in hockey coverage and one of the top guys on the whole Triple Crown coverage? I'm not quite sure I'm that smart. But I knew this guy was going to go into broadcasting after his career ended. There was definitely a career for him.

I developed a kidney stone early in the new year. Anybody who has ever had a kidney stone will tell you it's pretty painful. We talked to the Rangers and they suggested going to the hospital, where they tried to break up the stones with electrical shock waves. It took a few days but I passed the stones and, believe me, it felt like rocks when I eventually passed them. I felt like a landscaper with all those stones.

Around this time, Tommy had the chicken pox. So, it was quite an eventful time for us all, and Diana was in her last trimester. She drove to the hospital, dropped me off at the emergency entrance, then went home.

But things were about to get even more complicated.

CHAPTER 10

Good-bye, New York; Hello, Winnipeg (Again)

WE ALL KNEW MIKE KEENAN wasn't coming back to coach the Rangers, which was a whole other distraction for us during the Cup run. Keenan and his agent were talking with the Red Wings about becoming their next coach, even though Keenan denied everything.

On July 14, one month after we won the Cup, Keenan resigned. Two days later, the St. Louis Blues announced they had signed him to a multi-year contract as general manager/head coach. There was a whole lot of drama the way it unfolded.

Keenan and his lawyer claimed the Rangers materially breached his contract by not paying him a bonus he was owed, which they said allowed him to sign with another team. The Rangers filed a lawsuit with the National Hockey League a few days before he resigned, claiming Keenan had a binding deal and could not sign with another team. It was left up to NHL commissioner Gary Bettman to sort it out. He ordered the Rangers to pay Keenan $608,000 in bonus money and, in turn, he had to pay the team $400,000. Commissioner Bettman prevented Keenan from starting the job for 60 days. He was also fined $100,000 for conduct detrimental to the league. The commissioner also fined St. Louis $250,000 and Detroit $25,000, respectively, for tampering while Keenan was still under contract. The fines for Keenan and the Blues were the maximum under league bylaws. As compensation for signing Keenan while he was still under contract, the Blues traded young center Petr Nedved to the Rangers for left winger Esa Tikkanen and defenseman Doug Lidster.

If it would have been a player, assistant coach, or somebody like me who was an extra during the Stanley Cup run negotiating with another team, our names would have been tarnished for the rest of our careers. Keenan would have been front and center as part of the parade route ripping me or anybody who did that. But he did it. And how many jobs did he take and get fired after that? For everything that he preached and talked about how you can't be selfish and everything is about the team and everything is about the guys in the room, he was the complete opposite if you looked at some of the stunts he pulled.

A month later, the Rangers named Colin Campbell the new coach. My thought was, at least I'm going to get a chance to play. We had also lost a bunch of players, so just by default I'd be playing more. I had a good training camp and preseason, scoring three goals in one game.

And then came the lockout.

On January 11, the 103-day lockout ended. The NHLPA refused to accept a salary cap, but agreed to a rookie salary cap and changes to the arbitration system. The schedule was reduced from 84 games to 48, running from January 20 to May 3, and restricted games to conference play. That meant the Western Conference teams and Eastern Conference teams didn't play one another, which significantly reduced travel. During the lockout, a bunch of us on the Rangers worked out and played shinny a couple of times a week at the team's practice rink in Rye. Rye Playland is where the movie *Big* with Tom Hanks was filmed.

We played Buffalo in the season opener and had our championship banner–raising ceremony and it was awesome. John Davidson of the

MSG Network was the emcee and he introduced Rangers greats Rod Gilbert and Ed Giacomin, who walked on to the ice to participate in the ceremony. That was followed by a video of the goal Stephane Matteau scored in double overtime to win the conference championship. The camera panned to Matty and you could see he was awed, and the video included Howie Rose's epic call—"Matteau, Matteau, Matteau!" Then the Eastern Conference championship banner was raised accompanied by some blaring jazz music. Five longtime season-ticket holders were brought on to the ice as a tribute to all Rangers fans. A video showed the last seconds of our Cup win and the mad celebration that ensued on the ice and Mess letting fans touch the Cup. Another video was shown, this one of Neil Smith's comments at the Cup ceremony in which he thanked all our fans, whom he said were the greatest in the world and how we won it for them. It was followed by a clip of Adam Graves saying, "The bottom line is Rangers fans and the people of New York will never, ever, ever have to hear '1940' again."

We were gathered in a circle around center ice, the lights were dimmed, and the Cup was lowered from the rafters with the symphonic sound of "O Fortuna" from *Carmina Burana* and flashing strobe lights. Then the Stanley Cup banner was raised accompanied by "Ode to Joy." Mess took the Cup and we all skated around him with the fans chanting "Let's Go Rangers" and the blaring music of Tina Turner's song "Simply the Best." After Steve Larmer accepted the Cup from Jay Wells, he skated a bit and then handed it off to me. It was incredibly amazing. I thought, will this be the last time I do this?

I certainly didn't think so at the time. Do I think about being a part of a team again and hoisting the Cup again? Every day.

The only thing that spoiled the evening was that we lost 2–1.

On February 7, we celebrated the birth of our third child, Alexandra. After boys dominated both our families and having two of our own, I think Diana and I were definitely hoping for a girl. Because I was named after my dad and Diana had the same name as my mother, I had suggested the name Diana if it was a girl. I thought it would be cool to have three Eddies and three Dianas—my mother, Diana, and our daughter—but that got the thumbs down.

I've been lucky enough to have been around for the delivery of all four kids and it's an amazing experience. Sometimes because of a job like mine, that is not always possible.

* * *

After 20 games, I had two goals and an assist, and then I received a call from Rangers GM Neil Smith. Diana answered the phone.

"Hi, it's Neil Smith, is Eddie there?" he said.

"Yeah, right," Diana said, and hung up the phone.

It rang again.

"Don't hang up, it really is Neil Smith."

Most hockey guys are ball busters and like to play jokes on each other.

Neil told me I was going home. I thought he meant Chicago, but he was referring to Winnipeg. The Rangers received a fifth-round selection in the 1995 NHL draft in return. Neil said rather than seeing me suffer as a spare part, he decided to trade me, especially because John Paddock, who was the coach when I last played in Winnipeg, was now the team's general manager and wanted me. I will be forever grateful to Neil for trying to restart my career.

John was a gentleman and I respected him, but I had to prove myself to coach Terry Simpson. Terry had coached the New York Islanders from 1986–87 partly into the 1988–89 season. After working as an assistant for the Jets from 1990–91 through 1992–93, he was hired as Philadelphia's coach for the 1993–94 season. He took over from John Paddock for the remaining 15 games of the 1994–95 season.

I called Assiniboia Downs' race caller Darren Dunn—Double D—and told him I was coming back to Winnipeg.

It really felt like I hadn't left. I was just so comfortable there. John was one of the best coaches I had played for; he knew what I could and couldn't do. He believed that I could get back to being a productive player, and when you have people who believe in you, you're willing to go through a wall for them.

Look, we enjoyed our time in New York, but to get a chance to go back to Winnipeg and play just felt right. Diana came and visited a couple of times and then we all moved to Winnipeg, living on the same street as before—Shoreline Drive in a suburb called Linden Woods.

I finished with two goals and eight assists in 13 games, and even though we didn't make it into the playoffs I liked our team and had high hopes for the next season. But Simpson wanted to go with younger guys and I sat out the first five regular season games the next year as a healthy scratch. I got back into the lineup and played a few games and then suffered a rib injury and was cleared to play but became a healthy scratch again.

It really weighed on me mentally. I walked through the garage door into the house and suddenly it hit me. It couldn't get any lower. I had an emotional breakdown in front of Diana, wondering how much more I could take. It was like, enough is enough. I wasn't one of Terry Simpson's guys but all I wanted was an opportunity. You get to a point in your life where sometimes you wonder, is it really worth putting yourself through this? You've been a go-to guy for most of your career and then you go a couple of years where you're not even in the lineup and then you're banged up and the coach doesn't want to put you in there. I kind of felt the ground was falling out from under me. A coach can yell at you, scream obscenities, embarrass you, call you out in the media, and you just kind of live with it. But when you're not allowed to play or you're not playing, that's when it really hurts. When you're not playing or getting an opportunity to play, you start thinking that you're done or that you really can't play. Once I hit rock bottom, I knew if I was given a chance to play again I was going to stick it to Simpson and prove to him that that he screwed up by not having me in the lineup.

Diana supported me as a sounding board and told me that she knew I was a good player and that I could produce. That's what relationships are all about; knowing what to say and how to say it and knowing when to be rough and when to be soft. Sometimes you need a release. You don't want to put that burden on your teammates. I had many conversations with my agent, Ronnie Salcer, and he never wavered. He always knew that I could play, be effective, and carry out my role regardless of what it was. When you trust people, you're able to share stuff with them. If you're going to ask them something or tell them something, you know you're going to have to be prepared for what's going to come your way. Don't tell me what I want to hear; tell me what I need to hear. It wasn't easy for Diana because I came home with my work, and as much as you try not to show your frustration, it's there in your body language.

Once I did get back in the lineup I was put on a line with Keith Tkachuk and Teemu Selanne and I started to score regularly. You're right: I should have been scoring playing with those two guys.

I scored a goal and an assist in a 5–3 win over New Jersey on December 29. It was the last game my future NBC broadcast partner Doc Emrick called in Winnipeg, not knowing if he and, more importantly, the Jets would ever come back.

This was an emotionally painful time to play for the Jets because we knew it would be the team's last year in Winnipeg. The Jets were going to be sold because the cost of running the franchise became too much. All teams pay players in American dollars, and with the Canadian dollar trading at 68 cents USD, it was particularly tough on the ownership of Canadian teams. We thought that the year before there was a chance the franchise would be on the move, but then everything fell through and the team was coming back for one more season. Now we knew it was just a matter of where more than when.

The people in Winnipeg treated me and my family just like the first time we were there and we became a permanent fabric in the community, spending 11 months of the year there. It's not like it is today, where players have two or three houses, and as soon as the season's over they get the hell out of Dodge. This is where our kids went to school and played sports. This was truly our home.

DIANA OLCZYK
Eddie's wife
Winnipeg was great. It was family oriented. He loved Winnipeg. We both did. He wanted to bring the Cup back to the city.

I finished the season with 49 points in 51 games, totalling 16 power-play goals and 18 power-play points, which I felt good about considering I was a healthy scratch early in the season. It was disappointing that we didn't qualify for the playoffs.

The team had a special night at the arena to say good-bye to the fans and thank them for their support. A handful of members from our team spoke, including me. I can't imagine what it must have been like as a young fan having my favorite team just get up and leave town. It was hard to talk to friends we got to know in the city, knowing they were Jets fans and wondering if the NHL would ever bring the franchise back to the city. To this day we still talk about when the team left. Thank God that it is back now and flourishing.

That rally was a way to let people know how appreciative we were for their support and we wouldn't forget them.

When I spoke I said, "We will always be Winnipeg Jets, and wherever the team ends up...and when it wins the Stanley Cup, it's coming back to Winnipeg."

It was emotionally hard to say that, but the fans went wild and it's something I will always remember. In fact, Google "Ed Olczyk Speech: Bringing Cup Back to Winnipeg" if you want to listen to it. (But please don't call me Ed. Just saying.)

DARREN DUNN
Assiniboia Downs CEO
That's another reason he is so beloved in this city. That was one of the most iconic Jets speeches ever. What really stands out is he really, genuinely wanted to play here. We went through a period in this town where a lot of folks weren't too keen on playing here. But here's a guy who loved Winnipeg and who was happy to be here.

The franchise shifted to Phoenix on July 1 and was renamed the Coyotes. I became a free agent that summer, but we didn't have any dialogue with the new ownership and management. I thought there was a chance I would go to Arizona, but the organization had other ideas. I heard through the grapevine the new ownership group didn't like my speech at the rally. Too bad—that was their loss.

CHAPTER 11

FROM L.A.
TO THE BURGH

BECAUSE I WAS A FREE AGENT after the 1995–96 season, I had a chance to decide where to play next. My agent, Ronnie Salcer, had some offers, but the Los Angeles Kings showed the most interest.

The Kings were going through a transition after the Wayne Gretzky era. He had been traded in February to St. Louis, ending his time in Los Angeles, which began with the historic trade that sent him from the Edmonton Oilers to the Kings in 1988. Many of the players who were part of that Gretzky era, such as Jari Kurri, Marty McSorley, Rick Tocchet, Tony Granato, and Kelly Hrudey, were also gone after the 1995–96 season. The Kings didn't make it to the postseason and the roster was overhauled by general manager Sam McMaster.

But the team was up and coming with some really good players, including defenseman Rob Blake; forwards Ray Ferraro, and Kevin Stevens; goalies Stephane Fiset and Byron Dafoe; and young players such as Yanic Perreault and Mattias Norstrom. The Kings were looking for a center and we thought it would be a really good fit and a chance to play for coach Larry Robinson, so we agreed to a two-year deal. It was a chance to get some security and get my skates back under me again. Ronnie knew the situation really well because he was living in Manhattan Beach and had a couple of his clients on the team.

One of the big differences about playing in Los Angeles was the weather. In my final year in Winnipeg, there were 17 days in the month of February in which the temperature was minus-40. It was brutal. Every day in L.A., the sun is out. And, yes, Hollywood Park and Santa Anita racetracks were in the area. Hollywood Park was actually right across from the L.A. Forum, the home of the Kings and Lakers.

Diana was seven months pregnant when we got to L.A. and on October 3, the night before our first game, she went into labor. We rushed her to Cedars-Sinai Hospital and it looked like she was going to have the baby the next morning. I called the Kings and told them I wasn't coming to practice because Diana was in labor, but I planned to be at the game—kind of like the scenario in Toronto but with a much different result. Things slowed down, but at 5:23 PM Diana gave birth to our fourth child, Nicholas.

Nicky came into this world and I said to Diana, "Okay, I gotta go. I'll be back after the game. Wish me luck."

I jumped in my car at about 5:45 and hoped to be at the arena in time for the start of the game at 7:30. Amazingly, it only took me about an hour to get from the hospital to the Forum. I walked into the rink wearing flip flops, shorts, and a T-shirt because I didn't have time to change into a suit.

We were playing the New York Islanders, and in the second period while we were on a power play I won a faceoff, went to the front of the net, and redirected the puck and scored my first goal as a King. I got the puck and kept it. It turned out to be the only goal of the game.

After the game, I got back in the car and drove to the hospital to see Diana and Nick.

So that was my welcome to L.A. story. Ray Ferraro, who was one of my teammates and whom I played with quite a lot, remembers me rushing to the rink and scoring the goal. He says it's not like I needed any more energy, but I was pretty energetic that day.

We were renting a house in what is considered Beverly Hills—zip code 90210, like in the TV show—but in the lower-rent district. Our team's practice facility was maybe 20-25 minutes away. You'd see some stars every once in a while, at the dry cleaners or at the racetrack. My wife and mother remember running into Ringo Starr at a craft store. When you are talking about one of the Beatles, that's pretty salty air. There were a lot of movie stars who would come to the games and you'd cross paths with them every once in a while, but I would say Ringo would probably be the one that sticks out for our family.

I felt secure with the Kings and we were really enjoying our time in L.A. It was great on and off the ice.

I bought an unraced filly thoroughbred called Dialit Up with a group that included Ronnie Salcer and some of my teammates, including Kevin "Artie" Stevens and Rob Blake. Dialit Up was trained by Chris Baker, who had worked as an assistant to Richard Mandella and Neil Drysdale, two of the top trainers in the world. I believe Dialit Up was the first horse Chris trained, but unfortunately it didn't work out. Ray Ferraro ribbed me, suggesting I should sell the horse to somebody in New York to ride around Central Park and give carriage rides to get our money back. We did end up selling the horse. Recalling that time, Ray says he didn't realize how passionate I was about horses and that it was an education for him about my interest away from the rink. Chris Baker, incidentally, is now the chief operating officer for Three Chimneys, a major commercial breeding farm in Kentucky.

Artie started calling me Edzo, with that unique Massachusetts accent of his. I had no idea why Artie called me that, but it would turn out to be a nickname that would become more prominent later in my life.

Okay, time to tell a few funny L.A. stories.

First one, we were at our pregame meal at the hotel and I was sitting next to Artie, who was my roommate. We got on the topic of college athletes being paid under the table and everyone became involved in the conversation. Artie played college hockey. Ray Ferraro, who played Canadian Major Junior hockey, was chiming in from another table.

I said I had heard a story or two where players would go to sponsors' homes for dinner over the course of a hockey season and after the players had picked up their plate and taken it to the kitchen to be washed, there would be an envelope under the plate.

Kevin Stevens stopped dead in his tracks and said, "Edzo, that's a stupid thing. That doesn't happen."

I said, "Artie, it happens."

So now we're the only two arguing in the room and everyone is listening. We start going back and forth and he's telling me I don't know anything since I never went to college because I turned pro after playing in the 1984 Olympics.

So once again he said, "Edzo, you're stupid."

I said, "Artie, don't call me stupid."

"What did you say?"

"You heard me."

As I got up to get something to eat, he said, "Edzo, stupid, stupid, stupid."

There is this wooden soup ladle at the buffet and I walked up behind him and smashed the soup ladle right in his back. Artie's 6-foot-3 and 230 pounds. The soup ladle wasn't going to do anything, but I was so pissed off at him because he had hit a nerve calling me stupid.

Meanwhile, guys were roaring.

"Edzo, what are you doing?" he said. "I didn't mean like you're 'stupid' stupid. I meant like you're goofy stupid. There's a difference."

I got so mad I walked back up to the room and I grabbed the pillow from his bed and the ironing board from the closet and a glass of water and I laid it out right in front of the door and locked the door.

Ten minutes later Artie is trying to get in the room and says, "Edzo, don't be mad. I just thought you were goofy. I didn't mean you were stupid."

"Artie, tell me you're sorry," I said.

"I'm not telling you I'm sorry."

"Then you're not getting in the room."

"All right, I'm sorry."

"Tell me you love me."

"Edzo, there are people out here."

"Artie, you're not getting in the room until you tell me you love me."

"Okay, Edzo, I love you. You're sensitive. I didn't mean you're stupid. You're goofy when you talk sometimes."

I finally unlocked the door and let him back in his room.

That's the type of story you can't make up.

Here's another one. Our team was on a flight and some of the guys were playing cards. Somehow, we got to talking about playing craps, but nobody knew how to play. I said that I did, so they asked me to explain it.

"It's kind of hard to tell you," I said. "You need a table. I've got the dice."

They couldn't believe I had dice on me.

I went to the back of the plane and asked for a cardboard beer box and I got a couple of markers and I drew up a craps table. I brought the craps table back and put it on the floor and the card game stopped. I started explaining the Xs and Os of craps—craps for dummies, no pun intended—and we had a little game of craps 30,000 feet in the air.

Ray Ferraro remembers that story, but I think he was more amazed I had the dice in my bag than that I knew how to shoot craps.

Okay, I have one more. We were flying from Dallas to L.A. in January, the worst time for the Santa Ana winds. The pilot said, "I've got good news and bad news. The bad news is LAX is closed all day because of winds. The good news is if we can't land in L.A., we're going to have to stay in Las Vegas for the night."

We take off and the plane ride is a little bumpy.

Full disclosure, I've been known to be a bad flyer. Everybody chimes in, "All right, Edzo, this is it, kiss your ass good-bye."

I'm sweating bullets. The plane ride is getting pretty rough and there's dead silence. From the back of the plane, Dougie Zmolek, one of our defensemen, yells up to our general manager Sam McMaster, "Hey, Sam, sign the pilot, he's got more balls than half the guys on this plane."

Sure enough we have one of the worst landings ever. We would have had a better chance in a Pepsi can than we did in that airplane. We were bouncing around, dropping up and down, and when we got off the plane I actually had to walk with my head down to get through the wind because it was so strong.

RAY FERRARO
Eddie's teammate

Kai Nurminen was a first-year player, maybe 26 or 27, who had come over from Finland, and he was a little unsure of the whole league. It was a big move for him. This one game he got hit and was out with a bit of a thigh injury. Eddie picks up on this right away and starts calling him Thigh instead of Kai. Kai kept correcting him, thinking Eddie didn't know his name. He'd say, "It's Kai," and Eddie would say, "Okay, Thigh," just to have some fun.

So we were playing a game and I had the puck and Kai was yelling for it. I didn't know where I was on the ice. We go back to the bench and Kai says, in his Finnish accent, "Ray, did you not see me? I was three meters behind you." Eddie, who was on our line, is cracking up as I said, "Kai, how far back is three meters?" We were just dying because he was trying to tell me he was about 10 feet away, but we didn't know how far that was.

We just thought that was hilarious. We weren't a very good team, but we had a lot of fun.

* * *

Things were going well for me. I scored a hat trick in a game at home against Vancouver that we won 6–2. I had 13 goals at that point of the season. I was playing again and getting plenty of ice time.

The trade deadline was March 18 but I wasn't expecting to be moved. Practice had been pushed back that day to 2:00 PM local time, a couple of hours after the deadline. I was at home and at about 12:10 our time, my buddy Dominic Porro, who was in town visiting from Chicago, blurts out, "Trade deadline is over. You're not going to get traded."

Within about 30 seconds the phone rang, but I didn't think anything of it, so I just picked it up. Sam McMaster was on the line and he told me I had been traded to Pittsburgh for forward Glen Murray. Way to go, Dom.

Diana was on her way home from the doctor with Nicky, who had his six-month checkup, and I kept looking out the front window for her. I wasn't looking forward to telling her because I knew what her reaction would be. The house that we lived in was kind of at the top of the hill, so I went outside and I could see her in the Town & Country a couple of hundred yards away. Eddie and Tommy were in school and I was home with Zandra.

I was outside standing where the sidewalk connected with the driveway, and as soon as Diana pulled up into the driveway she looked at me and didn't even stop. The garage was maybe another 30 feet away, but somehow, she knew I had been traded. I could see that by the look on her face. When she got out of the car, she was pretty angry. She handed me Nicky and started crying and ran into the house. It was just one of those things where you feel helpless. She had been through a lot physically and now she had to deal with this, knowing I was going to be away and she was going to have to look after the four kids. It wasn't going to be easy but we'd get through it somehow.

To this day, I blame Dominic for being the kiss of death.

This was one trade that really caught me off guard. There were no rumors or speculation, and then the next thing you know I got the call. We were only there for six months, but we were treated well and made some lasting relationships. I loved L.A.

I wish it would have worked out a little better. I really enjoyed playing for Larry, who was a great teacher of the game. We underachieved that year, and at the time of the trade had a record of 25–37–9. So, on the one hand it was hard for me personally, but professionally it was good because I was going to the Penguins.

Pittsburgh had a record of 32–30–7 and was headed to the playoffs. The team had made a recent coaching change with general manager Craig Patrick taking over on an interim basis from Eddie Johnston. I knew Craig from my days with Team USA in the Olympics and the Canada Cup.

The Pens had Mario Lemieux, Jaromir Jagr, Ronnie Francis, and Joey Mullen on their star-studded roster and they were looking for some added scoring depth for the stretch run and the playoffs. Pittsburgh had won the Stanley Cup in 1991 and '92, so it wasn't all that bad joining the Penguins. And they had some of the best trainers ever. Sev, Pauly, Little Pauly, Scotty, Johnny, Guru—I love those guys. I have been very lucky in my career. I have gotten along with all the trainers I have had as a player or coach.

Initially, it's pretty breathtaking and intimidating being on the same team as Mario. We came into the league together in 1984, and if I had chosen to play in the Quebec Major Junior Hockey League I would have been on the same team as Mario. So here I was all these years later and finally getting a chance to play on the same team as Mario. He was such an imposing figure, but it turned out great. What an experience. I ended up rooming on road trips with Ronnie Francis, who is still one of my closest friends. He's a man's man, class like you wouldn't believe. Ronnie is the same guy now as he was as a Hall of Fame center or later as the GM of the Carolina Hurricanes, which he should still be, by the way. (He had a great assistant GM as well: my brother Rick.) He is a great man, a mentor, and a great family man. I am lucky our paths crossed.

Mario had been through so much with missing the 1994–95 season battling non-Hodgkin's lymphoma and back problems. Just to try to see him get ready to play, let alone seeing him go out there and perform, was pretty inspiring. It was also hard to watch because he was taping himself together just to get out on the ice. He needed help to tie up his skates but once he got the blades on, it was phenomenal. To lace them up and go out there and be one of the best players on the ice—a guy that could barely bend over—that was pretty inspiring.

Mario and I developed a friendship. We had a Masters pool on an airplane trip not long after I was traded and all the guys on the team drafted players in the tournament. I had read an article on golfer Willie Wood indicating he might have a long shot chance to win the tournament. There was a whole production with these pools, similar to the NHL draft in which a team announces it is proud to pick a particular player. In this case, it was, "Eddie Olczyk's team is proud to select, with the 55th pick, Willie Wood." Being a golf aficionado, Mario thought it was the greatest thing and kept repeating "Willie Wood, Willie Wood." He'd call me Willie and I'd call him Willie and they became nicknames that continue to this day. Willie Wood tied for 12th that year at one-under. A pretty good selection, I might say, 17 shots back of Tiger Woods. It was fun stuff. I'm not sure whatever happened to Willie Wood, but my friend Willie helped save the Penguins from leaving Pittsburgh a few times. Way to go, Willie!

Time for one more funny story, and this one involves the Kings again. They were flying in from L.A. to play us on March 29, my first game against them since I had been traded. They arrived the day before the game and I happened to get some steam on a horse in the sixth race at Santa Anita. I was going to meet Artie and Ray at an off-track betting shop and then go out for dinner. They landed in Pittsburgh, went to the hotel, dropped their stuff off, and took a cab to the Ladbrokes OTB in Moon Township, right near the airport.

I told them they had to get there before the race went off, although I said I would bet a few bucks for them. It was two minutes to post and they still hadn't shown up. Sure enough, they came in with the horses on the way to the gate.

I said, "Just tell the teller you want the 10-horse to win in the sixth race at Santa Anita." Artie and I bet with both hands on that one. We all made a nice score. It was well worth the aggravation of getting from the airport to the hotel to the OTB. Incidentally, we won the game 4–1 and I had a goal, my first with the Pens.

Initially, I played a couple of shifts with Mario and Jagr, then I played with Ronnie for a period of time, and then Tyler Wright and Alex Hicks. I was up and down the lineup. Craig told me I could be playing with Mario or I could help the fourth line, so I just had to be prepared with whomever and whenever. In 12 games, I scored four goals with seven assists.

We finished second in the Northeast Division with 84 points and faced Philadelphia, which finished in the Atlantic Division with 103 points and second overall in the Eastern Conference, in the opening round of the playoffs. Mario led our team in goals (50), assists (72), and total points (122) in the regular season. He won the league's scoring title for the second consecutive season. He said before the playoffs began he would be retiring after the playoffs ended because he felt he couldn't play at a high level anymore.

I played with Tyler and Alex in the playoffs and we were considered the energy line. Philadelphia won the first three games, but we won the fourth game in which I scored a shorthanded goal. Philadelphia ended the series in the fifth game. It was disappointing not be able to go that far in the playoffs knowing the Penguins' history.

Mario scored three goals and three assists in the series and had a goal and an assist in the final game. He had battled and tried everything he could possibly do to play but he just wasn't comfortable. Any time you see a legend step away because of health reasons or an injury, that's hard. It was a culture shock for everybody and, in addition to that, the franchise was not exactly on stable ground financially. It was a changing of the guard, for sure.

Ronnie Francis took over as captain of the team after Mario retired. Craig Patrick hired Kevin Constantine, who had coached San Jose from 1993–94 through the first 25 games in 1995–96. He was a guy who enjoyed having the authority, playing a lot of mind games to see how players would react in certain situations. He was kind of like Keenan. Constantine wasn't a popular guy, but coaches don't have to be popular. You just have to produce.

That next season, I scored nine goals and totaled 12 points in my first 20 games, missing a few with a minor injury. In my 23rd game of the season, I broke my zygomatic arch, or cheekbone, taking a puck off of my face on a shot from teammate Fredrik Olausson. I ended up playing only 56 games that season, scoring 11 goals and adding 11 assists.

One of the funniest things happened the morning after we played a game. Eddie was playing a game for the Mt. Lebanon Hornets at Mt. Lebanon Ice Arena—the same place I got initiated as a rookie with the Hawks—and Tommy was sitting next to me. One of the referees was trying to be like an NHL referee, calling icing and offsides like a hawk.

I was a little tired and agitated, and I was starting to get angry because the referee was taking control of this game with six- and seven-year-olds. There's no flow to the game and the referee, who's probably in his late 30s or early 40s, calls an intentional offside on these kids. There's maybe 55 parents in the rink. These kids don't know their right shoe from their left shoe and this guy's calling an intentional offside?

"Come on, ref, what do you think this is, the NHL?" I yell out. "Let the kids play."

As he was going down to the other end for the faceoff, I see him turn back and look at me. I'm about 25 yards away and he blows his whistle and yells, "You, out."

What is this guy doing? He's throwing me out?

Kathy Galloway, the manager for our team, came over and said, "We can't start the game until you leave the rink."

I was sitting with my son Tommy and as we were leaving the stands, he asked me, "Are you going to tell Mom?"

I walked to the back of the rink and watched from the back wall. I was punished and had to go in the timeout corner and watch the rest of the game. It wasn't the last time I yelled at an amateur referee but it was the first and only time I have been thrown out of one of my kids' games.

The Penguins finished first in the Northeast Division with 98 points and second overall in the conference behind New Jersey, which had 107 points. We played Montreal, which finished fourth in the division, in the opening round. We lost the opening game 3–2 in overtime but won the second game 4–1. I scored the opening goal on the power play. We lost the third game 3–1 but won the next game 6–3. I scored my second goal of the playoffs in this game, this time on the penalty kill. We lost the fifth game 5–2 and the series ended in Game 6 with Montreal winning 3–0.

The season was over. I was a free agent, again.

CHAPTER 12

FAREWELL, HOCKEY

I WAS HOPING TO get a chance to come back to Chicago and play one more time for the Blackhawks, and that's exactly what happened. General manager Bob Murray, who was a teammate of mine when I broke into the National Hockey League, offered me a one-year contract. Bob Pulford, who had played such a huge role in my career, was still with the club as senior vice president of hockey operations.

So much had happened since I began with the Hawks in 1984, so it felt like I had come full circle. Unlike when I joined the Hawks the first time, there was no announcement or press conference when I re-signed. There also wasn't the pressure I put on myself when I was a rookie. I was much more mature and experienced and had been around the block. I was just looking for an opportunity to play and make the best of it. I don't think Diana and I ever suggested to the kids this was likely going to be the end of my career.

Things did not start the way I envisioned. I was a healthy scratch early in the season, so the team sent me down to the minors to play for the Chicago Wolves of the International Hockey League. Believe it or not, my first practice with the Wolves was in the rink where I grew up playing hockey, the Ballard Sports Complex in Niles, Illinois. I started playing the great game of hockey on this ice when I was six, and here I was again all these years later. During that first practice I thought, is this it? Will I ever get back to the show after playing hockey for 25 years? Am I at the end? Will this be the place I skate for the last time?

BOB PULFORD
Blackhawks senior vice president of hockey operations
We brought him back because we thought he could help the hockey team. We felt he was a top player. He was a good person and I was very proud of his success. I was happy for him.

Kevin Cheveldayoff, who is now the general manager of the Winnipeg Jets, was our general manager with the Wolves at the time and he was incredible in the way he treated me. I am thankful to Chevy for taking me on his team. He knew I wanted to get back to the NHL and gave me an opportunity to play. John Anderson was the coach and I had known him from his days playing in Toronto, Quebec, and Hartford.

I think my first game as a minor-leaguer with the Wolves was in Winnipeg against the Winnipeg Moose. That whole experience was just kind of surreal, being in the Peg, where I had some incredible nights as a Jet, and now here I was in the minors.

There was a scrum around the net and there were five or six guys pushing and punching. All of a sudden, this guy from the Moose grabs me from behind—I have no idea who any of these guys are on either team—and he was getting a tad aggressive as we separated a bit from the pile of players. We finally got face to face and he had this look like he wanted to drop the gloves.

Allow me to digress. For the record, I did fight the late Bob Probert when I was with Toronto and Probie was with the Detroit Red Wings. Okay, I did a lot of holding on—I was no dummy—and the official NHL box score lists both of us getting five minutes for fighting. So, there you go.

But back to the face-to-face encounter with the Moose. This kid said, "You want to go?" So I said, "Hey, kid, I am not sure who you are, but I know Zinger [Craig Heisinger, the Moose's GM and my equipment manager in Winnipeg for more than five years] and if you don't take your hands off of me and leave me alone, I will tell him to trade you."

He smiled and politely took his hands off of me. The kid was Jimmy Roy and he told Zinger that story the next day and he got a huge chuckle. To this day, anytime I see Zinger we still talk about that story.

I got called up to the Blackhawks around Thanksgiving after seven games in the minors. The team made a coaching change after 59 games with our record 16–35–8, replacing Dirk Graham with assistant head coach Lorne Molleken, someone who would figure prominently in my life a few years later. Lorne had played in five minor leagues over the course of his pro career from 1976–77 through 1984–85. He began his coaching career in the Western Hockey League, starting out in 1988–89 for three seasons as an assistant with the Moose Jaw Warriors. Then he became head coach of the WHL's Saskatoon Blades for four seasons. After that he worked in the American Hockey League as a head coach for one year with the Cape Breton Oilers and two years with the Hamilton Bulldogs. He was in his first season as Dirk's assistant when he was appointed head coach. Lorney was to the point, supportive, and understood guys' strengths and weaknesses. A great guy and a really good coach.

I played on a line with Tony Amonte and Alex Zhamnov for a lot of that year and finished with 10 goals and 15 assists in 61 games. I signed another one-year contract after that.

In the summer of 1999, Dominic and I played the Illinois Mega Millions, a twice-weekly lottery in which you pick five main numbers and a Mega Ball number. The game offers jackpots starting at $40 million. Frequently, the jackpot rolls over into hundreds of millions because no one has a winning ticket.

We had played it various times in the past, but this time there was an $80 million jackpot. We played about $300 worth of tickets, using both automatically generated numbers and some we selected ourselves.

The drawing took place the night of July 23 and the winning numbers were 6, 10, 24, 26, 37, and 6.

We were off by one single number.

Dominic called me the next morning, thinking that at least we had won a consolation prize of $250,000 because we had five of six numbers correctly, but it was actually only $5,000. Nothing to sneeze at but not $80 million. The one number we missed was 24. We had 23.

No one had a winning ticket and the jackpot the following week was $150 million.

When I think of beating the odds, that would have been the ultimate case financially.

Right from the start of the 1999–2000 season, I was bothered by a herniated disc, although I tried to play through it. I played five games and then one morning I woke up and pretty much just had no feeling in my right leg. I couldn't stand up and knew I had to get it fixed. I had surgery in the middle of October and returned to the lineup about two months later.

With our team struggling and a record of 5–13–4–2, Bob Pulford replaced Lorne, who became his assistant. Pully was the best coach I ever played for back when my career began and here he was coaching me again, although Lorne was running a lot of the day-to-day practices and I developed a great relationship with him.

I returned to the lineup for the 32nd game of the season and was basically in and out of the lineup thereafter. After I played on March 24, I didn't see any game action and was just skating to stay in shape and trying to get healthy. Prior to the last game, which was at home, Lorne talked to me and said he knew I wanted to play next season, but the team wouldn't be offering me another contract. He said it would probably be a good idea if I thought about playing in that last game, but I told him I didn't want any handouts. He said I'd earned the opportunity to play in it and if I chose not to do it I might never get an opportunity to play in the league again. He also said if I elected not to play in that final game, I'd always wish that I had. I emphasized I didn't want to do it, but he asked me again to think about it.

I didn't want to feel like I was playing for the sake of playing. I went home and I talked to Diana about it. I also called my dad. They both said I should play, that if the team wants me to play and I'm healthy enough, I should do it.

I went to practice the next day and told Lorne I would play and he was very happy. He reiterated that I had earned the opportunity and privilege to play one last time as a Blackhawk. Listening to Lorne was one of the smartest things I ever did. The organization gave me an award as Man of the Year for my community service before the game started. It was really hard, very emotional. I think there are photos of me sobbing accepting this award, knowing that was going to be my final game as a Hawk and possibly the last game in my career. Thanks, Lorney. I got the Tomahawk Award, which is given to the player of the game, by my teammates and kept it. I still have it in my house.

DIANA OLCZYK
Eddie's mother

The last game was emotional. I felt the cheers. It was like, this is the end. After each hockey season, it was like a sadness and I couldn't wait for the next season to come. This was the ultimate end. I knew he loved playing hockey so much.

LORNE MOLLEKEN
Eddie's coach

Eddie was one of our leaders. He was the type of player at the end of his career that I thought I could put into a lot of different situations. One time we had our goalie pulled and we needed a goal to tie the game and I sent Eddie out to take a faceoff against Mark Messier. Eddie won the draw and we scored. Bob Pulford looked and me and said, "Why would you put Olczyk out there?" I said, "Well, he won the faceoff." He was the type of player who left everything on the ice. He wore his heart on his sleeve. It was a pleasure coaching him.

The Hawks had hired Mike Smith as manager of hockey operations four months previously. The last time I had any contact with him was during the arbitration for my contract with the New York Rangers going into the 1993–94 season. So here we are about seven years later at my exit meeting and he asked me what I planned to do. I said I still might want to play and he said it wasn't going to be with the Hawks. I asked if I could retire a Blackhawk and he said the team only did that for good players. I wasn't asking for a press conference; I was just looking for a chance to say thank you to the organization and the fans, but he wasn't going to let me do that. I think he was still pissed off because of what happened in the arbitration.

I had a conversation with Oilers GM Kevin Lowe, who was my teammate on the Rangers team that won the Cup in 1994, about possibly signing with the Oilers, but I decided I didn't want to uproot my family again. I retired a couple of months later.

Similar to my signing the second time around with the Hawks, there was no formal announcement. After 16 seasons, my NHL playing career was over.

CHAPTER 13

A NEW PERSPECTIVE

FOR YEARS, I HAD THOUGHT about what I would do when my career ended. I had no idea when it would happen, but I was already thinking about a second career. Would I be a coach? A broadcaster? An agent? Or just chase my kids around the country as their lives played out? It was all on the table.

For many athletes, regardless of the sport, it is not an easy transition. You become accustomed to a set routine as a player, in which you are given a schedule to follow, and all of the sudden that is taken away. Now you have to think about what you will do with your life. How will you make a living? How will it impact your family?

I needed some advice, so I called John McDonough, who was the senior vice president of marketing and broadcasting for the Chicago Cubs. Our paths crossed over the years; he grew up in the same area of Chicago as I did. I wanted to get his take on the options I had pursuing a TV broadcasting career. I had been doing some radio and TV broadcast work during the last few years of my playing career.

John proved to be an incredible resource and took the time to give me some advice on what I should do. I explained to him that the Hawks' TV analyst spot was open, but I did not get the gig. I told John about the opportunity I had to go to Pittsburgh and become the TV analyst of the Penguins with Hockey Hall of Famer Mike Lange. I will be forever grateful to John for taking my call. I did not know it at the time, but our paths would cross again seven years later when John would become my boss as president of the Blackhawks. It is truly a small world.

JOHN McDONOUGH
Blackhawks president and CEO

Being a Chicagoan, he called and asked me for some advice. I remember walking around Wrigley Field with him. Nobody was there. I told him if this opportunity presents itself with the Blackhawks, pursue it. He had every characteristic to succeed, all the intangibles. I didn't know then that he and Doc Emrick would basically be the face of hockey in the NHL. But I'm not at all surprised with his success. He's just got this unique personality that people gravitate toward.

DIANA OLCZYK
Eddie's mother

I prayed to God, believe me when I tell you this and God gets the glory and the praise, and said, "Please, get Eddie a job in broadcasting." I kid you not. I just thought he'd be perfect for it because he sounded good on the radio and he knew what he was talking about.

I decided to take the gig and commuted between Pittsburgh and Chicago for the next three years. There's no doubt working as a hockey broadcaster helped ease the transition away from playing the game. I was still traveling with a team but with a lot less pressure. I lived at the home of a former teammate of mine, Ronnie Francis, for the first two years in the burbs of Pittsburgh because he was playing for the Carolina Hurricanes. Ronnie is the man, none better. He is classy, respectful, and a great landlord, too. The price was right for living in his place. The only time I angered Ronnie and his wife, Mary Lou, as the tenant was leaving the garage door open one day. Minus one on Edzo. It never happened again.

I had a lot more free time back home in Chicago on days off. I could take the kids to school or to hockey. When I was playing full time, I did what I could do. Everything was built around my schedule and Diana had to do a lot of the heavy lifting, but once I stopped playing I became available more.

Mike Lange is just an incredible guy, a legend, an icon in Pittsburgh. He had been the team's radio and TV announcer since 1976 and had become known to fans for his interesting and colorful descriptions, which became known as Lange-isms. His body of work earned him a place in the Hockey Hall of Fame as the recipient of the Foster Hewitt Memorial Award for outstanding work as an NHL broadcaster in 2001. I have been fortunate throughout my broadcasting career to work with so many greats and, in the case of Mikey, he was an incredible resource and influence. He took the time to give me some advice on how I could become a better broadcaster. He taught me about the business and preparation. We just had so much fun together, on and off the air. I wish there was a camera rolling when we were off air.

When you are a local broadcast team, you are catering to a certain demographic and fan base, and Mikey helped me so much. He's a big reason I was able to cultivate a broadcasting career, taking the time to help me along and critique me and tell me when I made good points. He had lots of time for me. I'd like to think we had fun together. He made me laugh all the time, regardless of what it was. Things may not have been going well for the team and I'd tell the fans to sit in another chair or go in another room to watch or turn your jersey inside out, and Mikey would just go on a laughing spree. It's great when you respect and love somebody like that who knows how to press your buttons. Working with Mikey is a big reason why I am where I am today as a broadcaster. I have so much love and respect for him and was fortunate to be able to work next to him for three years. He really helped mold my style.

MIKE LANGE
Eddie's broadcast partner
I was just absolutely stunned at his ability to handle the TV situation. I worked with a lot of people and Edzo came in and automatically knew what was going on. In our business, you have to listen to a producer talk in your ear. A lot of things are going on and he absolutely nailed it immediately. He was aware of time, he was aware of the situation. I had never seen it before and I haven't seen it after as far as somebody with that ability. I've told him, he's going to get into the Hockey Hall of Fame, but it isn't going to be as a player. It's going to be as a broadcaster. Edzo will do that before it's all done.

One thing I learned in my transformation to full-time broadcaster is, it's not what you say, it's how you say it. The job is to tell people why things happen and what will happen. I played with hundreds of guys in my career—is it hard to call them out when they make a bad play? Yeah, sure it is. I don't have a reputation of railroading guys or making it personal or holding a grudge against somebody.

The telestrator and learning how to use it that year became a big part of my career and I credit that to the great production people working at Fox Sports Pittsburgh with me. It's a great teaching tool to take people inside the game, whether they know hockey or not, and I got to do that in Pittsburgh. In any walk of life, success is partly based on how you separate yourself from everybody else, and the telestrator became part of my repertoire. It was being used in the broadcast industry as a regular thing. John Madden was doing it for NFL games and back in the day Howie Meeker used it for NHL games. There is a cost involved in using it, with wiring and cabling and all that kind of stuff. I started circling people in the crowd for fun—kind of like highlighting a play—and it soon caught on. People started bringing signs that said CIRCLE ME EDZO, an homage to the Tickle Me Elmo doll that was very popular at the time.

One of the most interesting things that happened early in that first season was Mario Lemieux coming back to play and ending his three-year retirement. He was training in the dark and I was among five retired players who were asked to skate with him so he could get some company on the ice and practice shooting on a goalie. The trainers were ordering a bunch of sticks for him, and you're not going to deny 66. When I watched him skating and shooting and saw he was in great shape, it was clear he was on his way back.

Adding a guy like Mario, regardless of how long he had been out, made the team that much better. Yes, he was the owner, but he was also one of the greatest players in the history of the game, and if he thought he could help put the team over the top, it made sense. Why not? He owned the team.

I had only been retired for eight months and I missed playing. Mario's comeback made me wonder: if I could get back into shape, would there be a spot on the team for me? Coming off of a back injury, I didn't know if I could physically do it. But I never talked to anybody about coming out of retirement and after skating for a couple of months, it never went any further than that. Even Diana didn't know.

Mario made his return in Pittsburgh on December 27 against Toronto and the game was televised nationally in the United States and Canada on separate networks. It was a huge story. The crowd went wild when he stepped on to the ice before the game began, many holding up signs. There was a sign in the crowd that read HEY SANTA, THANKS.

"Being a former player, you get that feeling that you don't appreciate something until it's gone and it's great to have Mario back," I said on the broadcast.

In typical fashion, Mario assisted on the game's opening goal by Jaromir Jagr at 33 seconds of the first period. Mario threw a pass out in front of the net and Jagr scooped it in. The play was reviewed and I used the telestrator to show how the goal was scored. The crowd erupted when Mario's name was announced for assisting on it. Mario scored a goal midway through the second period on a one-timer from the slot on an excellent cross-ice pass from Jagr.

"He is smiling like a butcher's dog," Mike said of Mario.

"Was there ever any doubt?" I replied. "You know where to score goals, and even after a three-year layoff, you never lose that feeling."

Mario added another assist in what became a 5–0 win. That game was one of those surreal things that further underlined he was superhuman, just an amazing athlete. The team had a record of 15–14–6 and one overtime loss going into the game and won three in a row after Mario's return. He had nine goals and 12 assists in his first 10 games and the team had six wins. It was a circus atmosphere everywhere we went because of Mario's comeback. So, in my first year out of the game, I got to see a legend end his retirement and look as good as ever. It was spectacular.

Mario finished the season with 35 goals and 41 assists in 43 games, almost averaging two points a game. Think about those numbers. He had 16 power-play goals and 32 power-play points. The team finished with a record of 42 wins, 28 losses, nine ties, and three overtime losses. To put that in perspective, the team basically tripled its win total with him in the lineup.

The Penguins opened the playoffs against Washington and won the series in six games, and Mario had four goals. They faced Buffalo in the division final and won the first two games and then lost the next three. But they won the next two games, both 3–2 overtime victories. Mario had two goals in the series. The Penguins faced New Jersey in the conference final, but lost in five. Mario finished with six goals and 11 assists in the playoffs. It was a hell of a run for him and the team.

But it didn't last.

The team traded Jaromir Jagr in the off-season as part of a cost-cutting move, and following an 0–4 start head coach Ivan Hlinka was replaced by Rick Kehoe. Mario only played 24 games, and when it became apparent the team wouldn't make it into the postseason, some of the key players were traded. The team finished last in the division.

After finishing last again the following season, Rick Kehoe was relieved of his duties, along with the team's minor league coaches. It was not known who would replace Rick.

It turned out to be me.

CHAPTER 14

BEHIND THE BENCH, BRIEFLY

IN THE FINAL FEW YEARS of my playing career, I began thinking about a career in coaching. Flat out, I wanted to stay involved in the game. As a player, I had been a go-to guy, a high draft choice, and a Black Ace. I played on the top line and the fourth line—in every role. I had been a part of a team that won the Stanley Cup. And I had played for every type of coach imaginable. I loved the teaching part, the fixing, and watching the guys enjoy the rewards of executing and winning.

I was a student of the game. I liked to get an edge on players, particularly goalies, and on what teams were doing or what tendencies they may have had. I'd make notes and put them down on paper. When I got traded to Toronto in 1987 we lived in downtown Toronto at Bay and Bloor—400 to be exact. The next year we bought a house in the suburb of Unionville and I bought a satellite dish for the house so I could watch as many games as possible and do a little scouting as well. I also found some time to watch some horse racing on the dish; a great investment, I may say. I would set the VCR and record my games so I could scout myself, too. I'd watch the game, but fast forward to my shifts to see what I did and didn't do.

But I wasn't just watching my games. I'd watch every game I could. That's how much I was into hockey—and still am. But you also have to remember that when I began my career, there were no subscriber packages such as NHL Network or Center Ice to watch every game. You were at the mercy of a satellite dish and you didn't have access to every game.

After broadcasting Penguins games for three years, I contacted Pens general manager Craig Patrick about the team's head coaching vacancy with its Wilkes-Barre/Scranton affiliate in the American Hockey League. Craig and I had a long history together in the USA Hockey program, both at the Olympic level and Canada Cup tournaments. He had been the head coach for the Penguins for the final 20 games of the 1996–97 season. We talked about my interest in applying for the Wilkes-Barre/Scranton job in our first meeting, an interview that lasted three hours or so.

Then we had a second meeting. This time he outlined what was going to be the plan with the Penguins. They were going to go with a really young team, move out players who still had value, and shed some cash. Winning was going to be tough and they were preparing for a work stoppage after the season because the Collective Bargaining Agreement between the owners and players was expiring. The organization wanted a young coach and Craig asked me if I would be interested in coaching the big club.

I went in for the minor league job and was offered the head coaching job of the Penguins. My mind was racing. What if I don't take it? What if I do? What will the hockey world say?

Speaking of that, I always found this to be hilarious. When I was named the head coach, some TV and newspaper hockey insiders north of the border ripped the decision: no experience, never coached, etc. All valid points, fair opinions, no issue there. But when the Great One, Wayne Gretzky, was named coach of the Phoenix Coyotes in 2005 with the same credentials as a head coach in the NHL as I had (which was about the only thing I ever had in common with No. 99), all I heard was the sound of crickets from those insiders. They took a holiday on their opinions. No plums, I get it. It's No. 99.

Diana and I had talked about my desire to coach. She looked at it one way, specifically the lack of security, but once I had the interviews with Craig my motor started running and I decided this was what I wanted to do. I talked to a select group of people I trusted—Ronnie Francis, Ronnie Salcer, and Lou Lamoriello were among them—asking their advice. I'd say 70 percent of them suggested I should take it, but there were some who thought I should decline because I had no prior coaching experience and the franchise was up in the air at that point. But ultimately the decision was up to me and my family.

On June 11, I was unveiled as the 18th head coach in Penguins history and the second-youngest head coach in the NHL at the time, five months older than the Carolina Hurricanes' Paul Maurice. It was emotional for me because I had not expected any of this when I originally spoke to Craig. It had all happened so fast. Yeah, I had no experience, but how do you get experience? You can either get it on the job as an assistant or straight into the role of head coach, and both Mario Lemieux and Craig felt I could handle it. Craig's first head coaching job was in the NHL with the New York Rangers in 1980–81 and the only experience he had in coaching was as an assistant to Herb Brooks with the 1980 U.S. Olympic team.

If you look at professional sports now, there are many examples of players who have gone directly into head coaching or managerial jobs without any previous experience. What kind of experience did Aaron Boone have when he was hired as manager of the New York Yankees? What about Steve Kerr before he coached the Golden State Warriors? Or Larry Bird with the Indiana Pacers?

The night before the official announcement, word leaked to the media. At the announcement, Craig told reporters that he knew there were probably going to be a lot of people skeptical of my hiring because

I had no bench experience. But he said there were many others who had jumped into the role of head coach without any experience and had done quite well. He referred to Terry O'Reilly, Brian Sutter, Bob Pulford, Gerry Cheevers, Glen Sather, and Al Arbour. He said he thought I would make a good head coach based on what he had seen when I played for the Penguins. He said I was more aware than anybody he'd ever seen as a hockey player of all parts of the game and I was like another set of eyes and ears, essentially another voice in the room. He said I had been very impressive as a broadcaster in analyzing, dissecting, and critiquing every move in every game, and became convinced after our conversations that I was a perfect fit for the job and he stopped talking to anybody else.

I told the media Craig knew what type of person I was and that I appreciated the opportunity and that it was an honor to not only represent the Penguins but also the city of Pittsburgh.

I inherited assistant coaches Randy Hillier, Joe Mullen, and Gilles Meloche from Rick Kehoe's staff, and I signed Lorne Molleken as my lead assistant because I respected him so much for how he coached and counseled me during his time with the Hawks at the tail end of my career. My biggest job was to sell hope, not only for that season but for down the road, too. I was our unofficial spokesperson and my message was we were going to have a lot of young players and we'd have to grind it out. But there's a difference between working hard and working smart. My plan was for the team to be relentless in creating offense, but at some point, your talent needs to take over to keep that going.

Overall, I was going to emphasize three things: communication, consistency, and discipline. I tried to mold myself with bits and pieces of coaches who had a positive impression on me, such as Bob Pulford, John Paddock, and Lorne. They were the three best coaches I ever had. I had some coaches who were at the other end of the spectrum, but you've got a job to do and if they tell you to play, you play. That's just the reality of it. You could learn from a bad experience or from coaches who saw you in a certain light. I was a go-to guy for a long time in my career, and then there were a handful of years where I was the whipping boy and a healthy scratch.

I helped Michel Therrien, who had coached Montreal for one full season and parts of two others, get the job in Wilkes-Barre/Scranton. I had known Michel through Denis Savard, who played for him, and we needed a tough coach in Wilkes-Barre/Scranton, and that's what Michel was. I told Craig that Michel had great experience and could be a resource for me.

In the draft, we selected goalie Marc-Andre Fleury first overall from the Cape Breton Screaming Eagles of the Quebec Major Junior Hockey League. Craig acquired the first overall selection after making a trade with the Florida Panthers, which had the top pick. Marc-Andre, nicknamed Flower because of his last name, became only the third goalie to be chosen first overall. Aside from Mario, who was the Penguins' top player the previous season with 28 goals and 91 points in 67 games, the lineup wouldn't have a lot of stars.

* * *

We opened the season at home and lost 3–0 to Los Angeles with Marc-Andre in net. He did his best, stopping 46 of 48 shots—the third goal was scored after we pulled him for an extra attacker. The following night in Philadelphia, we tied the Flyers 3–3, rebounding from a 3–0 deficit after the opening period. Mario had a goal and an assist. Five days later, we lost 4–1 in Montreal. I won my first game two days after that at home when we defeated Detroit 4–3. The Red Wings led 3–1 late in the second period, but we bounced back with three consecutive goals, including the game-winner by Rico Fata, who scored twice. He remembers I was so happy and thought it was because I fulfilled a spot in my life because I loved coaching. He also said he felt great to contribute and to be a part of that.

RICO FATA
Penguins player
When Eddie took over, the first thing that I really, really admired about him is that he called every single one of us in the summer time. He even called the Penguins [farmhands] in the American Hockey League. He called everyone that had an opportunity to make the team. I have nothing but unbelievable things to say about him as a human being. Those one and a half years in Pittsburgh with Eddie were my most memorable in the NHL. It was my most productive time and my most enjoyable time.

What I remember most about that game was a play I had been working on that I called Willie Wood, a reference to the nickname Mario and I called each other. In between the second and third period, I went to the dry erase board and got the team's attention with about five minutes left in the intermission. I turned to Mario and said, "Willie, your line starts. You win the faceoff and stay at the center dot and face our defenseman. Marty Straka and Konstantin Koltsov will circle under. You build up speed and change sides up the walls and while they are doing that our defense will pass the puck to each other. Then fire the puck at you, Willie, and all you do is redirect the hard pass from Dick Tarnstrom to Koltsy." As I was explaining and drawing the play on the board, I could see a lot of the guys looking at me like I was crazy. I continued with the plan, saying, "Chris Chelios is gonna run at you and all this open ice at their blueline will open. Tip it by Chelios and we will get a two on one and Koltsy will pass it to Marty and he will go top shelf and the game is tied."

We executed the play just as I had drawn up, verbatim. The guys and the trainers were all stunned. If I had a microphone in my hand, I would have dropped it. I felt like I was a coach after that.

I don't care what type of team you have, you want to win every game. But the longer it takes, the more you wonder if it's going to ever happen. When I did get that first win, I slept a little easier.

DIANA OLCZYK
Eddie's wife

When you're coaching and you're responsible for everything or you're in management, I think it's 24-7. For him it was 24-7 because he wanted to do such a good job for the Penguins. He wanted the Penguins to get out of this rut and get where they needed to be. He took it upon himself, for sure.

After 10 games, we had a record of 3–4–3. Mario didn't play another game that season because he was bothered by hip problems. We knew that Mario was going to be in and out of the lineup, so it was going to be a battle all season long because we didn't have a lot of scoring depth. After 20 games, we had a record of 5–10–4–1. Marc-Andre either started or played in a majority of those games and he was facing a lot of shots, many times 35 to 40 per game, sometimes even more, and he was starting to struggle. As an organization we made the decision to loan him to Team Canada for the 2004 World Junior Hockey Championships. We brought him back after the tournament, but ultimately made the decision to send him back to his junior team. He got a taste of the NHL playing in 21 games and had a record of 4–14, a goals-against average of 3.64, and a save percentage of .896. He was scheduled to receive a $3 million bonus if he appeared in 25 games and he was the best goalie we had in the organization, but finances were an issue and I totally agreed with the decision to return him to his junior team. We knew he was going to be a stud. What a great move by Craig and our staff to move up in the draft and get him.

CRAIG PATRICK
Penguins general manager
Marc-Andre had a bonus in his initial contract that if he played more than 25 games he got a huge bonus, so we could only play him 24 games. Eddie's right. We couldn't keep him the whole season and that did hurt us on the ice, for sure.

At the halfway point of the 82-game schedule, we had a record of 10–23–5–3.

The hardest part was about to come.

We went on an 18-game winless streak that stretched from January 13 until we snapped it with a 4–3 overtime win against Phoenix on February 25. Staying mentally focused throughout that and helping the team maintain that mindset was part of my job. We were thin in terms of talent to begin with, and once Mario stopped playing and we started trading guys away to cut payroll, we had a boatload of inexperience.

One of the greatest compliments I got was from Carolina's head coach Paul Maurice, who said our guys worked hard and had great structure. That's as good a compliment as you can get from another coach. People in Pittsburgh knew we didn't have a lot of talent and were looking to hit rock bottom, but the fan base was supportive, no issues whatsoever. The way it was going, we were going to get some top draft picks.

I had always taken the game home when I was playing and it wasn't any different when I was coaching. When you are playing five-card stud with three cards—and people could argue we only had two cards—sometimes you might be able to win with a pair of aces. I kind of knew the hand we had and focused on how to make our guys better. It wasn't going to be based on wins and losses. I had a job to do with those guys inside the room, and a lot of them didn't care about the three-year or five-year plan, and that was the hard thing. They wanted to win now.

We played some really good games during that stretch, but we didn't have any difference-makers, and you need a goalie to win you a game every once in a while. You can press all the right buttons, but if the guys don't go out there and cash in, it's going to be really difficult.

I just told the guys to stay with it and they did. It was not easy, but I tried to build them up and make them feel good about themselves, regardless of what their individual stats were or whether the team won or lost.

Rico says collectively the team was frustrated by the losing streak, but he admired that I stuck to the details, such as continuing with our power-play and penalty-killing meetings, scouting the opposition, and motivating everyone with positive speeches. In his opinion, we started every game well, but lacked the experience and the mental focus to fight through adversity.

We had a record of 12–42–5–4 when we ended the streak and from that point forward we started to get rewarded for our hard work. We went on a roll and finished with the second-best record in the league in the final 20 games. Our final record was 23–47–8–4. Once we broke that streak in Arizona it helped a lot, and you want to see players rewarded when they play the right way. We didn't have a lot of proven skill or high talent, but our guys played hard. I felt good about our future knowing all the experience the kids were getting had started to pay dividends. There was a belief and confidence.

We beat Washington 4–3 in our season finale. Afterward I stepped on to the ice to address the crowd, which had started to become a regular practice in professional sports. It was heartwarming to see a fan displaying a sign that read THANK YOU, EDZO. YOU ARE OUR MVP. I thanked the fans for their support on behalf of Mario, Craig, the players, the coaches, and all the people behind the scenes such as the ticket sales staff, media relations staff, and training staff. I said the one thing I was most proud of was we stuck to the plan outlined by Mario and Craig of playing our young players from the start of the season all the way to the end. I also thanked the Penguins organization for making my family and me feel part of Pittsburgh again. I stressed how much our team needed the support of the fans and the sponsors and concluded by saying hopefully in a year's time we'd be playing in the first game of the playoffs.

Lorne left after the season when he was offered the job as GM/coach of the Regina Pats of the Western Hockey League. Still, I felt our future was bright.

* * *

With the CBA ending, no one knew for sure whether or not there would be a work stoppage the next season. I had been through a few of them already, so it was nothing new for me, except this time I would be experiencing it from a different perspective. NHL commissioner Gary Bettman claimed the league and many teams were losing money because 76 percent of gross revenues were tied to player salaries. The owners wanted cost certainty with a salary cap, but NHLPA executive director Bob Goodenow disputed that.

In an *Associated Press* story, Mario provided his opinion on it. "A few years ago, I thought the owners were making a lot of money and were hiding some under the table, but then I got on [the owners'] side and saw losses the league was accumulating," he said.

I was going back and forth between Pittsburgh and Wilkes-Barre/Scranton because I was watching the minor league team play. While Wilkes-Barre/Scranton coach Michel Therrien and I spent some time talking about things, there was never a plan to have me working full time with the team. My role was pretty much scouting.

I spent some of my time helping coach Eddie, Tommy, and Nicky's minor hockey teams. They were affiliated with the Pittsburgh Predators, who played out of the Ice Castle Arena in Castle Shannon, about seven miles south of Pittsburgh. The Predators organization was started by Ralph Murovich and managed by his wife, Darlene. Their son Tyler played hockey with my boys. I had an open invitation to come out and help assist in the coaching. There were some youth coaches over the years who didn't want any help from me, some who wanted a lot of help, and some who wanted very little. I always respected their position. I had helped out the year before, but not as much as this time. I traveled with the team on road trips and it was a lot of fun. During the three years I was commuting back and forth while I was broadcasting, I had helped coach my sons' teams. Matt Bartkowski, a Pittsburgh native who played in the NHL for nine seasons as a defenseman, was on that team. John Moore, a defenseman with the Boston Bruins, was another kid who I helped coach as a player in Chicago. Tommy played with Johnny. In a November 2018 interview with Tim Wharnsby on the NHLPA website, John credited me with having an impact on his career when I coached him. "It was unbelievable to have him as a coach. You're so drawn to everything he would say because of his knowledge and passion for the game. It's something I feel fortunate and grateful for," he said.

When I was coaching the Predators, I was using the same teaching fundamentals and systems as I did with the Penguins. Take the schemes out of it and a lot of it is simple, basic fundamentals and reminders of what the hell is going on in a game or pointing out where to angle where the puck is coming off your stick blade for a pass, or pushing the puck instead of stickhandling. Yeah, I got my fill of coaching from that part of it and I loved working with those young kids, but it really didn't seem like going from the NHL to a midget youth team in Pittsburgh. I was also helping out Nick's squirt team. I didn't have a lot of free time, but I was catching up on missed opportunities over the course of the tail end of my career. Eddie and Tommy were playing high school hockey, so I was doing a lot of driving to practices and games.

The lockout stretched out from days to weeks to months. Every day I woke up thinking that day was going to be the day the work stoppage ended. There were all kinds of rumors and speculation and it was like a roller coaster. One of the rumors was that Mario Lemieux and Wayne

Gretzky, who was the managing partner of the Phoenix Coyotes, had come up with a plan, but it proved to be untrue.

On February 16, Gary Bettman canceled the season, making the NHL the first North American pro sports league to lose an entire season because of a labor dispute.

Did I think we were going to lose the whole season? Not in a million years.

On July 22, the NHL announced a six-year agreement had been reached with the NHLPA, which provided cost certainty. Player costs would not exceed 54 percent of league revenues in the first year but that could rise to 57 percent if league revenues exceeded $2.7 billion. Team salaries could be as low as $21.5 million and as high as $39 million. The minimum salary rose from $185,000 to $450,000. Additionally, there would be an entry-level salary for rookies, with the potential for bonuses based on specific goals and points, and an agreement by the NHL to participate in the Olympic Games in 2006 and 2010.

Because the season had been lost, it was decided a lottery system would be used to determine the draft order, based on teams' playoff appearances the last three seasons and first-overall draft picks from that span. Teams could have anywhere from one to three balls in the drum. We were among four teams with three balls, the Sabres, Blue Jackets, and Rangers being the others. Sidney Crosby, a center for Rimouski Oceanic of the Quebec Major Junior Hockey League, was considered a generational player similar to Mario. In fact, this was called the Crosby Sweepstakes. It was just a question of which team won the lottery.

I watched the drawing alone in my office. The top pick came down to Pittsburgh and Anaheim. Ken Sawyer, our team president, and Brian Burke, Anaheim's general manager, represented their respective teams. Gary Bettman announced the winning team and it was us. I heard a big yell in the hallway outside my office. Ted Black, who was the team's vice president, came into my office and gave me a big hug and a handshake. Then I got a call from Darren Dreger of TSN. He said, "Edzo, your job just got a little tougher." I never thought of it like that. I was just thinking we got the best player available and he's going to help get the franchise back to what it was in the early '90s. It was surreal.

After talking to Dregs, I went to the Penguins' youth hockey programs going on at the Ice Castle. There were probably 150 kids there and both the kids and their parents knew the results and were jacked. It was absolutely off the charts, just awesome. You just knew the team and the city were on the verge of something incredible.

Within a couple of days, things had changed significantly with the Penguins. Mario was thinking of coming out of retirement and all of a sudden, we found a money tree. Craig asked me to rate all the free agents and choose my top three, money not being an issue. The first name I gave him was center Mike Modano, who had played with the Dallas Stars. Modo's contract with Dallas had expired and we needed centers. It seemed like overnight the situation had gone from a season of rebuilding, going 18 games without a win but finishing with the second-best record in the league in the final 20 games; to drafting Evgeni Malkin but not having a season; to winning the lottery and drafting Sid; to finding money and deciding to become competitive. We had drafted Fleury, Malkin, and now Crosby—no brainer, no brainer, double no-brainer. We were going to go at this thing methodically, but with Mario coming back we needed better players. We were trying to go from the outhouse to the penthouse.

Modo re-signed with Dallas, so Craig made offensive defenseman Sergei Gonchar, who had scored 20-plus goals twice in his career, his top priority. He signed Gonchar to a five-year, $25 million deal. Scoring wingers Ziggy Palffy and John LeClair were also signed to multi-year, free-agent deals. Palffy and LeClair averaged 34.2 goals per season over the previous nine seasons. LeClair was nearing 400 career goals and had scored 50-plus goals three times in his career playing on the Legion of Doom Line with Philadelphia. Goalie Jocelyn Thibault was acquired in a trade. Add in Mario and Mark Recchi, a former 50-plus goal-scorer who had been signed in July 2004, and collectively there was a lot of scoring power. I also recommended free-agent goalie Curtis Joseph, but he opted for the Coyotes, who were going to be coached by Gretzky.

We went from a team with not a lot of talent to all of a sudden world-class talent, like going from 35 miles an hour to 75 miles an hour, from one extreme to the other.

Before the season began, the decision was made to send Fleury to the minors. It came down to money because the organization did not want to pay him his bonuses. Look, if you don't have goaltending, you've got no shot. He was our best goalie, but it was a business decision not to have him start the season with the team. We started out with Thibault and Sebastien Caron, who was entering his third season.

* * *

We opened on the road against New Jersey and lost 5–1. Two days later we lost 3–2 in a shootout against Carolina. We had Mario, Sid, and Palffy as shooters. Welcome to the NHL, Cam Ward. It was his first start in the league and he's facing those guys in a shootout, but none of them scored.

Then we lost our next three games, all in overtime—7–6 to Boston, 3–2 to Buffalo, and 6–5 to Philadelphia. Caron played in the loss to Boston. Fleury was recalled and played against Buffalo, stopping 38 of 41 shots. He and Caron played in the loss to Philadelphia. Fleury gave up four goals on 20 shots but rebounded in his next game, which we lost 3–1 to Tampa. We lost 6–3 to New Jersey in the seventh game when Thibault and Caron played. We lost 6–3 in Boston in our next game with Thibault in goal, facing 47 shots. The winless streak ran up to nine with a 4–3 overtime loss to Florida. We finally won our first game of the season against the Atlanta Thrashers 7–5.

So why did it take so long to get that first win? There are lots of reasons, but I'll believe until the day I die that if we'd let Marc-Andre

Fleury be our goalie to start the season, things would have been much different. But that's just my feeling. He was the best goalie in the organization; all the players knew it. Losing those games in overtime and the shootout were tough, but you've got to find a way to win and obviously we didn't.

What was apparent from day one was that Sidney Crosby was going to be a superstar. His work ethic and desire were off the charts. What made the greatest impression on me was his skating. He could get up and go and knew what he needed to do. I started him on the wing to remove some of his defensive responsibilities. Eventually I moved him back to center and let him play and live with whatever happened. You are trying to spread the wealth up and down the lineup, but you knew he was going to be a dominant center.

After that first 10-game stretch, we won four of our next nine games and then something crazy happened in the 20th game. We were playing the Flyers in Philadelphia and Fleury was with the team as the backup, but was going to be sent down to the minors because Philadelphia is near Wilkes-Barre/Scranton. In warmups, right wing Konstantin Koltsov hit Thibault in the throat. I was in the coaches' office and our head of media relations, Keith Wehner, who is a close friend to this day, came into my office and said, "Edzo, I've got good news and bad news. The bad news is Thibault got hit with the puck in the throat on a shot by Koltsy and is on his way to the hospital. The good news is the kid's got to play."

Fleury played and we won 3–2 in overtime on a goal by Sid, his ninth of the season. Fleury was out of his mind, stopping 45 of 47 shots. We had a record of 6–8–6 after 20 games after starting out our first 10 games 1–4–5. We were on a roll.

After the game I begged Craig Patrick to let me keep Fleury, but he said we couldn't for financial reasons. I had to pull Fleury into the office after the game and tell him he was going down to Wilkes-Barre/Scranton after beating the Flyers 15 minutes earlier. I had many of those conversations because he would come and go a lot, but that was one where the kid played amazing. We had the Flyers at home three days later with a chance to go 7–8–6 and even though I tried like hell, Craig would not let me keep Fleury. It wasn't meant to be. We lost 6–3 to Philadelphia, and while we beat Washington 5–4 at home three days later, we went into a tailspin and lost six in a row. Thibault and Caron were the goalies for the first two losses, Fleury played in the next three, and Thibault was in for the last loss of the streak, 5–0 against Minnesota at home.

A couple of things happened during that period, one involving Mario and the other my daughter. On November 27, we were scheduled to play in Tampa Bay and Mario had some issues with his heart in the morning and he was really scared. Mario had experienced a rapid heartbeat during the summer and went through a series of tests, but doctors couldn't find anything wrong. On the day of the Tampa game, I spent several hours with him in his room in the hotel while he waited for his wife, Natalie, to fly in from Pittsburgh. We talked about everything—life, the team, golf, our kids—to pass the time. I just wanted to let him know that everything was going to be okay; that's what friends do. It was a pretty emotional day. I left for the game, which he missed. We lost 4–1, and Mario played in the next one two days later in Buffalo.

A short period later we were in New York and Diana contacted me to say she was rushing Zandra to Children's Hospital. Zandra, who was in the fifth grade at the time, had been in and out of the hospital for two months with digestive issues, but this time she had broken into a fever and they were running all kinds of tests to determine what caused the infection. They did a variety of scans and endoscopies and determined she was lactose intolerant and had gastric issues. Diana has had digestive issues, but they weren't sure if this was genetic.

I couldn't get a flight to Pittsburgh, so I rented a car and drove through a rainstorm. I got there around 4:00 AM. Whatever was happening with the team, her health was the most important thing to me. If your kids are not happy and healthy, you've got to prioritize. Mario and Craig were great about giving me the time to deal with it.

Zandra woke up in the hospital and she asked me what I was doing there. I'm sitting there crying like a baby and my daughter is telling me to go back because the players needed me. I talked to her and Diana wondering what to do. All I could think of was Zandra. We thought the temperature was a good thing because it proved something was wrong. We asked the doctor what to do and decided if I stayed around it might actually make her more upset. Like an idiot, I flew back to New York. That trip was like something out of a movie. We lost 2–1 to the Rangers.

We flew back for three games at home, finally ending a six-game winless streak with a 4–3 win over Colorado. Zandra's temperature came down and we brought her home. In the midst of all this, Mario had been hospitalized again because of his heart issues, which were diagnosed as a condition known as atrial fibrillation, which wasn't career or life threatening and could be treated with medication. We lost 3–1 in Detroit two days after the victory over Colorado and the next night lost 3–0 to St. Louis.

We flew home and the next day there were news reports that I was going to be fired. I saw it on Bob Pompeani's sports report on KDKA-TV in Pittsburgh. Then I received a phone call from TSN's Darren Dreger, who said he had heard some rumblings of a change and I told him I hadn't heard anything.

Shortly after 6:00 PM that day, Craig called me informing me I had been fired.

Was I expecting it? Well, considering all the rumors and everything else, you just think it's inevitable. I was expecting Craig to either knock on my door or I'd find something out the next day at practice. After he told me I'd been fired, I felt like I failed and let everybody down. I had a million things going through my mind. What could I have done differently? I just wished they would have given me Fleury for the whole year. That was my first thought.

Mario called me and I went to his home and had a face-to-face talk with him. He's the owner of the team and had a responsibility, but he was also my friend. We talked about how I appreciated the opportunity he had given me and his friendship. I wanted to clear the air and make sure he heard from me what I thought had taken place when he wasn't around because of his heart issue. When Mario was around, some guys were like church mice, and when he wasn't around, all of a sudden they became locker room lawyers and started flexing their muscles. There were certain veteran guys who rode the young guys hard in the locker room, but didn't take too kindly to it when they got put in their place. I am all for having young guys learn the ropes, but when it's personal, that's different. I came in during a hard era and had to earn my way. There were certain guys who were pricks to me as a player, but when it goes over the line that's where the coach or other veterans have to step in. If it would have happened when Mario was around, it would not have been accepted. But since it only happened when Mario wasn't around, that's when I thought it became a personal agenda and it was too much.

In an *Associated Press* story that ran the day after the firing, Craig said the 5–0 loss to Minnesota was "very disturbing." He said, "The team had shown its face and for whatever reason they weren't listening."

I don't think the team quit on me. I think a few vets quit on all of us! More than tuning me out, the team quit on the hand that was dealt and realized we had no chance of winning because the best goalie in the organization was not allowed to play. That's what I saw and felt.

LORNE MOLLEKEN
Eddie's assistant coach

When things weren't good and we were going through those long losing streaks, he shouldered all the weight. That takes an awful lot out of a person, and being a new coach and experiencing the losses piling up, he was just that type of person. He wanted to fix it. Coaching is very demanding and it took a toll on all of us. I thought he did a really good job. The players all respected him and liked him. Unfortunately, we just weren't very good at that time.

Sidney Crosby had some interesting comments about my firing in a story written by Shawna Richer in the *Globe and Mail*: "We're a family. When you lose a guy like that it's like losing people in your family. He was always there. He was the first one to take the blame and held himself responsible. As a player, it's not something you like to see. The coach doesn't put on his skates and go out and play. There's only so much he can do. I have a lot of respect for him. It's my first year, and coming in he communicated well with me, with us. He cared about us as a coach, especially me. I'm 18, and he gave me an opportunity to play here and I feel fortunate for that. It's tough, but sometimes hockey goes like that."

In an *Associated Press* story, Mario said, "Players are responsible for going on the ice and at least making an effort and, if you don't have that, it's difficult." He added that Therrien, who was going to take my place, is totally different. Look, Michel and I had two totally different philosophies on how to go about doing things. Obviously, Michel had a lot of experience and I had little.

Ryan Malone was quoted in an *Associated Press* article saying, "Losing is always depressing, but we've been embarrassing ourselves." That's

Bugsy's opinion and that was only his second season in the NHL. Was he right? How we were losing would probably play into that answer.

RONNIE SALCER
Eddie's agent

I think the timing might have been off. It's really tough to coach your contemporaries, and if you do you really need to get the help from the leadership, which I think Eddie relied on and that did not happen. It's really tough to execute your game plan when you don't have that and I think that was pretty much Eddie's downfall.

Look, the record speaks for itself, but like I said it's tough to win when you are playing five-card stud with three cards. That's the reality of it. You could put Joel Quenneville or Darryl Sutter behind the bench at the same time, and if you don't have a goalie, you are not going to win.

MIKE LANGE
Penguins broadcaster

The bottom line in this league is wins and losses. Unfortunately, he got into a situation where the team still wasn't really strong enough to be a competitive team on a daily basis. Sidney Crosby was here, but he was in his first year. They just didn't have the horses, to put it in his terms. They didn't have the ponies to make a clean run. There's a lot of demand for people wanting the team to win and changes and I think he got trapped in it.

But he knew that going in. He wasn't blind to it. I was disappointed he was let go, but you are hired to be fired in this business, unfortunately.

Craig decided to move up Fleury for the rest of the year and he played in 50 games, the most of the four goalies on the team, and he finished with a 3.25 goals-against average. He has become one of the best goalies of his era and will be a Hall of Famer when he retires. Would we have been better if Fleury was our starting goalie all the way through? You're goddamn right we would have been better. Maybe I would have been fired at the end of the year anyway, I don't know. But I don't care what anybody says, that decision had a major hand in where we were and how the team was performing.

I also wonder what would have happened if I had started out in Wilkes-Barre/Scranton and gained some coaching experience. The guy I recommend for the job in Wilkes-Barre Scranton replaced me, but that's just the way it goes—that's hockey.

I don't regret at all taking the job. I'm disappointed I wasn't able to see it through but not in a million years do I regret taking it. Yeah, it's easy to look back now and say I wish I'd had more coaching experience. Maybe it would have turned out differently. I'm sure Craig probably thinks the same thing. But who knows? A lot of things happened during my coaching tenure that were out of my hands, but I never regretted one bit taking Craig up on that opportunity. I did my best with what I had at my disposal. At the end of the day it's up to the coach to figure things out.

CRAIG PATRICK
Penguins general manager
It's hard to go back and project what may have happened in anybody's career. You just don't know. Circumstances are circumstances, and unfortunately, they don't always work out the way you want them to.

Mario returned to the lineup in the first game with Michel behind the bench and the team lost 4–3 in overtime. Fleury was in goal for that game, which turned out to be the last one of Mario's career. He retired a month later citing family, health, and an inability to play at the level that made him one of the greatest players in NHL history.

Mario and I had a great relationship through a span of eight years in which he had known me as a teammate, broadcaster, and coach. It didn't end on the greatest terms but that's business. Overall, there was a lot of respect on both sides. Willie took care of me and I hope he knows I tried to do the same.

On December 16, the day after the firing, Zandra said she felt fine for the first time in two months. When you have digestive issues, things like stress, lack of sleep, and diet can take their toll. There's no doubt in my mind she was feeling some of the stress that I was living with while coaching that team. If your children feed off and harbor that negative feeling, whether or not it's verbalized, it can make anybody ill. I considered it a fair trade-off, me being fired but my daughter getting her health back.

The team finished last in the division with a record of 22–46–14, including 14–29–8 with Michel. After the season, the organization opted to not renew Craig's contract. He was with the franchise almost 17 years.

CHAPTER 15

BACK TO THE BOOTH

AFTER THE SHOCK OF being fired, you're left with the emotional fallout. You've gone from being on a schedule and going 1,000 miles an hour to an abrupt halt. You're down, you're disappointed, you feel like you've let everybody down, and you're not sure what's going to happen. It's pretty traumatic when you've got nowhere to go in terms of work. It's a lot different than being traded, because at least then you know that while one team doesn't want you anymore, another one does, and you still have a job. Now the big question was, what do I do next?

In January 2006, Sam Flood, the coordinating producer of NBC Sports, flew to Pittsburgh and interviewed me about the possibility of joining their network hockey coverage as in-studio analyst. Sam played hockey at Williams College in Massachusetts and was captain in his senior year. He had been a freelancer with ABC Sports straight out of college when I played in the Olympics and had worked his way up to his current position.

We had dinner at Morton's Steakhouse in Pittsburgh and I felt pretty good about the conversation and that it was going to go somewhere. Did I think I would become NBC's lead hockey analyst or the lead handicapper of its horse racing coverage? No. But I felt something was going to materialize from that initial meeting with Sam because we hit it off right away. He subsequently hired me to do studio work for the NHL on NBC for the balance of the regular season and the playoffs.

In May, I received a call from Jimmy DeMaria, the executive director of communications, broadcasting, and community outreach for the Blackhawks, asking me if I would be interested in coming back to the organization to do TV color commentary for the next season on Comcast SportsNet Chicago.

I was exploring some assistant coaching options in the NHL and head coaching jobs in the American Hockey League, but this opportunity stood out among all the others. The chance to go back to Chicago and rejoin the Blackhawks organization was something my family and I simply couldn't pass up. After what I had gone through getting fired by the Penguins, I needed to do something. What an opportunity!

Blackhawks vice president Peter Wirtz said in a media release I had always been a Blackhawk at heart. He said I had a "very warm and engaging personality" and it was great to have me back in the organization working with the team's partners at Comcast SportsNet. The late James J. Corno, senior vice president/general manager for Comcast SportsNet Chicago, said the company was thrilled to have me working on the broadcasts because I was a local fan favorite and had truly done it all in the hockey industry. He said my uncanny knowledge of the game would be a tremendous asset to the telecasts.

Around this time, I received a call from USA Hockey offering me the chance to be the head coach of the U.S. team playing in the Hlinka Gretzy Cup, an under-18 world tournament in August in the Czech Republic. Jeff Blashill, who in later years became the head coach of the Detroit Red Wings, was chosen as my assistant.

To get that opportunity to represent my country again after playing in the Olympics, three Canada Cups, and four World Championships was very exciting. It was a chance to coach some future and current NHL stars such as Ryan McDonough, Cam Atkinson, and Jimmy Hayes.

Eddie, who had playing midget hockey with the Pittsburgh Predators, was also on the team. I had a say in the team, but USA Hockey had the final call. Eddie had a really good camp in the tryout for the team. The U.S. did not send its best players to the Ivan Hlinka tournament, whereas Canada did. Eddie was a fourth-line penalty-killer who knew his role, and because of that it wasn't a conflict for me giving him playing time. It wasn't even an issue. But to have that opportunity to coach the team and have Eddie there was a cool experience.

I had a lot of fun coaching the kids. We finished with a 3–0 record in the preliminary round, including beating the host country 4–3 in overtime in our last game, to finish atop our group. We qualified for the gold medal game against Canada, the tournament favorite. The Canadians also finished undefeated in the round-robin in their division. Unfortunately, we lost 3–0 to the Canadians, who outshot us 30–20. We had some good chances, but didn't have the bounce in our step that we had throughout the tournament and Canada played a really strong game. But I couldn't have been prouder of our players. It was USA Hockey's best finish in the tournament since 2003 when it won a gold medal after beating Russia.

* * *

I had assumed when I was hired to work on the Blackhawks games I was going to work with Pat Foley, who had been the team's longtime play-play-play man and the guy who I grew up listening to along with Dale Tallon. What a great broadcasting team. Pat had done play-by-play for the team full time from 1984–85 through 2005–06. I had no idea Pat was on his way out as I was coming back home. I remember calling Pat and sharing the news I was coming back—there was a pause on the other end—and then he shared with me that he wasn't going to be my partner and was on his way out of the booth.

Pat was replaced by Dan Kelly Jr., whose father was a legendary announcer with the St. Louis Blues and a Hockey Hall of Famer. Dan Jr.

had worked on HDNet's NHL coverage in its inaugural season the year before and had previous hockey broadcast experience doing TV work for the Columbus Blue Jackets and radio play-by-play for the St. Louis Blues. Those were very tough skates to fill for Danny. He was a great guy and a great partner. But you are really in a no-win situation when you are replacing a Chicago legend.

The Hawks finished fifth in the Central Division in the 2006–07 season, but won the lottery to select first in the upcoming draft. Dale Tallon, who was then the Hawks general manager, chose Patrick Kane, an offensively gifted right wing who had played junior hockey with the London Knights of the Ontario Hockey League. The native of Buffalo became the Hawks' first American-born player drafted first overall in franchise history.

Everybody knew Patrick Kane was going be a franchise player, a generational talent, somebody who would take the team back to the playoffs. But it's not easy to live up to the hype. It's a lot of pressure. Along with drafting center Jonathan Toews of the University of North Dakota third overall the previous season, the Hawks were starting to build with a new core of young players that also included defensemen Duncan Keith and Brent Seabrook.

The Hawks' hierarchy changed following the passing of Bill Wirtz in September 2007. Mr. Wirtz had built the organization and I will always be grateful to him for signing off on the decision to bring me back to Chicago to finish off my career. Mr. Wirtz and the entire Wirtz family have always treated me so well over the years regardless of where I was in my career.

A quick story about Mr. Wirtz. I was driving to Sioux City, Iowa, to watch my son Eddie play in the USHL for the Musketeers when my phone rang. The caller ID said "Mr. Wirtz's Office," and my first thought was, oh no, what did I do? I answered and Mr. Wirtz's secretary, Cindy, said he wanted to speak with me.

"Hey, Eddie, how you doing? Where are you?" he said.

After I told him where I was, he told me to drive safe and wished Eddie good luck in the game. Then he said, "I heard you're going to Las Vegas in a bit. I want to set you up. Dinner, shows, hotel, whatever you want, you got it. Just call this guy and you're all set."

Wow, what a gesture. I thanked him profusely. I knew the Wirtzes had connections out there thanks to their Breakthru Beverage Group operation. To this day, I have no idea how he knew I was going out to Vegas. I already had a room at the Red Rock Resort, but we jumped on everything else. It was a great trip.

That was Mr. Wirtz, no different than his son Rocky is today. Rocky always says, "If you ever need anything out there, let me know and we will take care of you." And the Wirtzes always have.

In October, Peter Wirtz left his position with the team, putting his brother, Rocky, in charge. Rocky decided to change the culture of the team, beginning with hiring Cubs president John McDonough to be president of the Blackhawks. John subsequently hired Jay Blunk, who had been the Cubs' senior vice president of marketing, as the Hawks' senior vice president of business operations.

Rocky made moves to turn around the franchise, which was struggling on and off the ice. In a nutshell, the team was in disarray. You had people in the office wearing four or five different hats. I'm sure there were a lot of things that were happening that we may never know about, but it had fallen on difficult times and wasn't very relevant in a great sports town. You could just tell Rocky, John, and Jay were going to do everything in their power to revitalize the Hawks. They started spending money and making the brand important. The Blackhawks were the last professional sports team to put all their games on television.

Under the new leadership, former Hawks greats such as Stan Mikita, Bobby Hull, and Tony Esposito were brought back as ambassadors. It helped reconnect the past with the present. Those players and this regime helped build the brand into what it has become. Rocky, John, and Jay showed they were going to do things their way and much differently than the past regime. They were going to mend whatever fences were broken.

My role with NBC changed after John Davidson, who worked as the analyst with Mike "Doc" Emrick, left in the off-season to become the president for the St. Louis Blues. Doc and I had worked together previously on NHL Radio. Being with Mike Lange, Doc Emrick, and Pat Foley, you are talking about three of the greatest play-by-play guys we've ever had in our game. It can be intimidating to be their broadcast partner. Mikey, Doc, and Pat are all perfectionists about their jobs, but it isn't life and death, and if you make a mistake you make fun of yourself. People love humility and all three of these guys have taught me that life is not easy and you're going to make mistakes. Yes, you want the broadcast to go well and not make any mistakes, but it's going to happen. As Doc says, "After a gaffe, oh well, it's off to Mars."

SAM FLOOD
NBC executive producer

He just seemed like a guy who had a lot of personality and a lot of passion. After John Davidson left it was a no-brainer that we wanted to move him into the booth next to Doc. Eddie was the clear first choice. We didn't look at anybody else.

There are plenty of broadcast teams that sadly have no relationship. They just do their jobs and get back on the bus. There's no camaraderie and no communication away from the broadcast booth. That would be really, really hard for me. The relationships that I have developed with my partners will be long-lasting. What I have with each of them is an incredible trust factor. We have each other's back and take care of each other on the broadcast and, more importantly, away from the booth. These guys are legends. It doesn't get any better than that.

On New Year's Day, I was part of NBC's broadcast of the inaugural NHL Winter Classic game played outdoors. It took place in Buffalo between the Sabres and Pittsburgh Penguins at Ralph Wilson Stadium and attracted a crowd of 71,217. We were outside on a scaffold behind the glass at the blueline across from the Penguins bench, about 15 yards from ice level and about 10 feet high. There were some complaints from fans behind us that they couldn't see the ice. But the idea was for us to be in the elements, which was something different. The wind became an issue being 10 feet above the ground as opposed to ice level, but the real challenge was losing some of the sightlines compared to calling it from the press box. There was also a glare from the lights that affected seeing the monitor. You're trying to do your job to the best of your ability but it was hard to sometimes see the players' numbers. For people watching on a high-definition TV, they're probably thinking, how could I not know that was Sidney Crosby or Colby Armstrong or Brooks Orpik or Jason Pominville? Look, we were just trying to survive. It was such a new and raw experience, but also exciting to broadcast. You had the face of the league, Sidney Crosby, and the Penguins, who were on the verge of taking the next step to glory. And you had Buffalo, which has always been a great market, on New Year's Day and it's snowing like crazy. Sabres goalie Ryan Miller wore a toque on top of his head. Collectively it had everything that the NHL, NBC, and fans wanted. And it had a great ending with the game tied 1–1 after overtime and requiring a shootout to determine the winner. Sid had a chance to win it, and Doc had recalled a game between Pittsburgh and Philadelphia in which Sidney was on a breakaway. His line in that game was, "The goal is on his stick." So, Doc used it again. Sid made a nifty move and beat Miller between the legs. You knew he was going to score because he's that type of guy. It was a storybook ending and an incredible experience overall.

Meanwhile, the Hawks showed significant signs of improvement. The team finished with 88 points in the 2007–08 season, just missing the playoffs, a 17-point improvement from the previous year. Patrick Kane led the team with 72 points, including 21 goals, and won the Calder Trophy as the NHL's Rookie of the Year. Left wing Patrick Sharp, playing in his second full season with the Hawks after he was acquired in a trade with Philadelphia during the 2005–06 season, finished second with 62 points. He almost doubled his point total from the year before and had 36 goals compared to 20 from his first full season in Chicago. Veteran center Robert Lang, who had played with me in Pittsburgh in the 1997–98 season, finished third in team scoring with 54 points. Jonathan Toews, playing in his rookie season, also had 54 points, including 24 goals. Defenseman Dustin Byfuglien, a 2003 draft choice who was converted from a defenseman into a winger, played his first full season and chipped in with 19 goals. Defensemen Duncan Keith and Brent Seabrook both showed improvement. Nikolai Khabibulin and Patrick Lalime split the goaltending duties. You could tell the team was on the verge of making a run.

For the start of the 2008–09 season, Pat Foley was brought back by John McDonough to do play-by-play after a two-year hiatus. That was part of a big process that changed the way people looked at the team and the game. It was another example of the organization doing the right thing in turning around the franchise on and off the ice. The Hawks received acclaim from fans, the NHL, other teams, and other leagues for what they did. People have called it a renaissance and that's the perfect way to describe it.

When I turned pro, Pat was calling my games, so we had an existing relationship. I was really fortunate when he was brought back and I became his broadcast partner. The same with working with Doc. I had always known Pat, heard his calls, and knew how respected he was. Both guys are incredibly fun to be around and super supportive.

At the start of the 2008–09 season, Jonathan Toews was given the captaincy at age 20, the third-youngest in history. The Hawks were aggressive in the free-agent market, signing defenseman Brian Campbell to an eight-year, $56.8 million contract, the largest in team history, and goalie Cristobal Huet to a four-year, $22.5 million deal.

In September, Dale Tallon signed Joel Quenneville as a scout. Joel had coached in St. Louis from 1996–97 through 2003–04 and the team made it to the playoffs seven of eight seasons. He won the Jack Adams Award as the top coach in the league when the Blues finished first overall in the league in 1999–2000. He joined the Colorado Avalanche, with whom he won a Stanley Cup ring as an assistant coach in 1996, from 2005–06 to 2007–08, advancing to the playoffs twice. He left the organization in May and you just knew he was the coach in waiting.

After taking only a point in their first three games, the Hawks beat Phoenix 4–1 at home. That's when Tallon fired Denis Savard as head coach and announced Joel as his replacement. At the press conference announcing the change, Dale said moving forward if the team wanted to be a championship-caliber organization, it had to make tough decisions and this was the toughest decision he ever had to make. Patrick Kane cried when he was interviewed, saying more than anything Denis was a friend. He said it was difficult to see him go, but hoped it would be for the best. Joel said the team was extremely entertaining and exciting with great youth and prospects for success. He said he was looking forward to fulfilling all of the objectives of being a top team and getting into the playoffs and going from there.

I felt bad for Savy, who was a great friend and had been with the team for a long time. He had coached the Hawks since midway in the 2006–07 season and had missed the playoffs both seasons. The team was on the verge of taking the next step and Savy deserved a lot of credit for helping mold some of those young guys into pros. Savy was a coach going through a rebuild, and next thing you know he's not the coach anymore and then the team goes on a run. I had experienced the same

197

thing. I'm sure Savy thinks about that all the time. But that's the nature of the beast and people get paid to make tough decisions that they think are best for the organization.

Right wing Marty Lapointe did an amazing job and helped a lot of these guys during his years in Chicago. With his experience playing eight seasons in Detroit, winning two Stanley Cups, and the way that he carried himself, he really helped set the stage for the guys inside that room to take the next step. That's one guy I always wish I would have had a chance to play with because he was so professional. I had the utmost respect playing against him for many, many years. Getting to know him in his time with the Hawks was a great eye-opener. My son Nick and Marty's son Guyot played youth hockey together one year. Marty made a huge impact with the Hawks, but was traded to Ottawa in February 2008. That's hockey.

The team was 4–4–3 after 10 games and then went on a four-game win streak. Beginning with the 25th game of the season, the team went on a nine-game win streak. It ended with a 4–0 loss on the second-to-last day of 2008 against Detroit. On New Year's Day, 2009, the Hawks played the Red Wings in the second NHL Outdoor Classic. This took place at Wrigley Field, home of the Chicago Cubs, and NBC broadcasted that game.

I had been to Wrigley hundreds and hundreds of times for baseball games, but seeing a hockey game played in the outfield was surreal. It was a crazy day because Doc had laryngitis and lost his voice the day before, so they brought in the late Dave Strader, the voice of the Phoenix Coyotes, who had broadcast NHL and Olympics games for NBC. I have a great picture of me and Strades doing that game. We had worked together on NHL Radio and ESPN prior to that Winter Classic.

It was a cold day—the temperature at game time was 27 degrees— and the wind was 30 miles per hour. It was like a wind tunnel. Bob Costas called it the friendly and frozen confines of Wrigley.

The Hawks were leading the league in attendance and this game sold out in an hour when it was announced, a capacity crowd of 40,818. This was another great "get" by the Blackhawks front office and a welcome home for John McDonough and Jay Blunk. It was the 701st meeting of the Hawks and Wings, the most of any of two teams in NHL history, and both teams wore retro jerseys. The crowd roared throughout the singing of the U.S. national anthem by Jim Cornelison, and fireworks went off during the "rocket's red glare" part. Toward the end two MiG jets flew above Wrigley.

Once again, we did the game from an area just outside of the glass at center ice. But the weather was far more cooperative than the year before. Pierre McGuire, who was dressed in a toque, gloves, jacket, track pants, and skates, did a pregame interview with Patrick Kane, who was wearing a balaclava and had eye black to battle the glare. Many of the players did the same thing. Patrick said the first time he was at Wrigley he threw out the opening pitch and sang "Take Me Out to the Ball Game." He added it was a pretty cool experience, almost like skating in an open field against one of the best teams in the world.

Darren Pang interviewed Red Wings defenseman Chris Chelios, who grew up in Chicago and was the NHL's oldest active player, playing in his 25th season. He joked that he'd never seen so many guys happy to go to practice the day before.

The game turned into a chippy affair with plenty of fisticuffs in the first period, a carryover from the game two days before. Dave noted there had been boxing at Wrigley Field in the past and now we had hockey players dropping their gloves and fighting.

The Hawks scored the opening goal, but lost 6–4 after giving up five unanswered. I remarked that it was all part of the process for Hawks. Overall, it was a lot of fun to be a part of broadcasting a game between two of the Original Six teams playing in the signature game of the NHL regular season at Wrigley. Doing a hockey game from the home of my favorite baseball team was both fun and awesome. Strades did a great job filling in for Doc.

Detroit finished first in the division with 51 wins, 21 losses, and 10 overtime losses for 112 points, followed by the Hawks with 46 wins, 24 losses, and 12 overtime losses for 104 points. The Hawks beat Calgary and Vancouver in the first two rounds of the playoffs, setting up the conference finals against Detroit. The Red Wings won the series in five games, but overall it was a great season of growth for Chicago. Martin Havlat led the team in the regular season with 77 points and in the playoffs with 15 points. Duncan Keith emerged as a solid two-way defenseman—I could see he was a future Norris Trophy winner—who had a plus-minus of plus-33. Jonathan Toews led the team in goals with 34. The Hawks were a young team and you knew they were on the verge of something. It was just a matter of time.

* * *

On June 18, the NHL Awards show took place in Las Vegas for the first time and I was there as a presenter and brought along Thomas as my guest. Any chance I get to handicap horse racing I take my shot, and I decided to take one at the Pick 6 at Hollywood Park in California because the pot was pretty big, about $500,000.

In a bet such as the Pick 6, where you have to pick the winners of six consecutive races, money management is almost as important as knowledge of handicapping. It costs a minimum of $2 to play, but it increases by the number of horses you play in each race. For example, if you bet three horses in the first race and two in the next, it costs $12. It can run up to hundreds and thousands of dollars if you play a whole slew of horses. The real secret is picking long shots that don't appear to have a chance, because if all the favorites or shorter-priced horses win, the more overall winning tickets there will be.

I didn't invest a lot of money, less than $200, and I had the first four winners and only needed to win the last two races in which I had three horses in each. There was a horse that was running for the first time after getting gelded—I know the feeling after being gelded myself after Nick was conceived—and I liked to use that angle if the horse had some decent form. Getting gelded is, as they say at the track, the ultimate equipment change. For whatever reason I didn't play that angle and the horse won. I ended up with five of six winners and there was a consolation prize for that. Even though I won a few grand, I was so pissed off because if I had used the gelding I could have won $400,000.

We left the next day to return home so I picked up the *Daily Racing Form* the night before to make my picks. We got to the airport and our flight was delayed a couple of hours because of weather issues. The first post time was 9:00 PM CST. I decided to wager $168. I called my son Nick and told him to tape the races on the TVG Network.

By the time we collected our bags and got home, it was a little after 11:00 and two races had already gone off. I watched the third leg live at home and I had only one horse, Streets of Heaven—my stone-cold single—trained by Neil French. I had no idea what the horse's price would be. The horse had run only a couple of good races, including one seven days before. He showed speed and French gave him a race to get fit—what's known as a tightener—and this time they would take the horse back off of the pace and let him make one run. I thought he'd maybe go off at 8-1, but he was actually almost 17-1. Jockey Alonso Quinonez grabbed hold of the horse and took him back in the field of 13. The pace was hot and the jockey was biding his time, waiting for one late run. Then he made his move and waded through traffic on the far turn and absolutely exploded down the stretch and won.

I went back and rewound the VCR and watched the first two legs of the Pick 6 and, yes, I won both races. So now I'm 3-for-3. I had the winners of the fourth and fifth races as well, and had seven of nine selected in the last race. I felt pretty good but didn't know how much it was going to pay.

It was probably midnight Chicago time and I'm super jacked. I called my buddy Dom, who was asleep and had no clue what was going on. I also called my buddy Joe the Judge, who's a big horseplayer, and my friend Coop, who lives in Ocean City, New Jersey. I also called Joel Quenneville, who is a horse owner and horseplayer. The first thing he said to me was, "Are you alive in the Pick 6?"

I told Joel the numbers of the seven horses and he said, "The 10 is the winner." I then informed my family about the situation and they came downstairs to watch the race with me. Of the seven horses I had, the cheapest payout was about $58,000. The biggest payout was about $1.5 million to four different horses; I had two of them.

The winning horse was indeed No. 10—Suances de Espana, ridden by Martin Pedroza, the second favorite in the field. There were three winning tickets in the pool, each worth $498,711.20. Including the consolation prize for picking five of six winners, I won more than $500,000.

After kicking myself for failing to win the Pick 6 the day before, it all turned out, thanks to Streets of Heaven. The Olczyk family had a massive celebration and all of a sudden, the kids started to sing. Diana said, "Now we're going to get a pool." No chance on the pool, I thought, but there obviously was a lot of excitement. Winning the Pick 6 reassured me of my handicapping, but you also need some luck. Sometimes the stars are aligned and sometimes you've got to take a chance. And I finally got even.

A little while later, I looked at my Xpressbet betting account on my computer waiting to see if the money from the Pick 6 had been deposited. I kept pressing the refresh button and then finally it showed the winning amount, less 25 percent taxed by the government, and I was like, "Holy Jesus."

Unlike lotteries, racetrack winnings are not publicized, so while my family and friends knew I'd won, it was otherwise a secret. About a month later I was in Winnipeg and a reporter, Kirk Penton of the *Winnipeg Sun*, heard I hit the Pick 6 and wrote about it and that's how it became public. "Every squirrel finds a nut every once in a while, so I just happened to get lucky," I said. "It's a tough enough game to pick a couple of winners, let alone six in a row. But sometimes the combinations come up right."

* * *

In September, Eddie accepted a partial scholarship to play hockey at the University of Massachusetts–Amherst. He had a couple of opportunities, but UMass was the one that kind of stuck out with him. It was pretty cool for him and all of us felt proud. Tommy followed him a couple of years later into college hockey, playing for Penn State, which was just beginning a Division I hockey program thanks to former alums Terry and Kim Pegula, the owners of the Buffalo Sabres and Buffalo Bills, who gifted a sum of $102 million to build an ice arena and finance the hockey programs.

In February 2010, the NHL took a break for the Olympics and it was my first time covering the Games as a TV broadcaster. I had some previous experience as a radio broadcaster, but it was much different this time. People always ask me what broadcasting the Olympics is like compared to playing in it. Nothing will ever top playing in it, but it's incredible and an honor to be there as a broadcaster. To be there in Vancouver 2010 was pretty cool because of the atmosphere in Canada. Everybody hoped for a gold medal game between the U.S. and Canada.

The Americans and Canadians played a really exciting game in the preliminary round. The U.S. won 5–3 and toward the end of the game I described it as "tremendously tremendous." Full disclosure, my buddy Dominic is a wordsmith—I say that with my tongue in my cheek—who has this incredible ability to come up with phrases and sayings. It's kind of a language that we have amongst ourselves and our family. He also says things like "indeed of the indeeders" and "the best of the bestess." Over the years "tremendously tremendous" kind of stuck in my brain. I would use that language at home sitting on my couch with Dom or my family.

I never thought about using it in a work environment; it just came out organically. The game was so good that I didn't think "tremendous" did it justice. I thought I might as well let everybody know this game had been tremendously tremendous. It got a boatload of feedback on social media and you can watch the clip on YouTube. I honestly didn't think it would get as much play as it did and it has become part of the hockey lexicon. I saw a billboard a couple of years ago for an alcohol beverage company and all it said was REFRESHINGLY REFRESHING. I'm sure there's some guru out there who came up with that, but I'm the one who introduced tremendously tremendous to the world. I will give Dom the primary assist on that.

MIKE "DOC" EMRICK
NBC broadcaster

As for the "tremendously tremendous," that's Eddie. On an international stage you don't want to be sterile. You want to show this is an incredible event with guys who only have these teammates every four years. I think emotion is wonderful, and rather than being all stoic and professional and cold, I think people relate to somebody that's actually caring and showing emotion and coming up with something like that. It never crossed my mind as being oddball or strange. I just thought it was a tremendous statement and kind of funny.

The gold medal game was exciting, too, with Sidney Crosby scoring the winning goal in OT, which was described as "the golden goal" by Chris Cuthbert on the CBC. Doc didn't say a word after the goal; he knew he didn't have to. Someone timed the silence as a minute and 40 seconds before Doc said, "Now come the handshakes."

The Hawks followed up on their impressive season from the year before and took it to another level, finishing first in the division with a franchise-record 112 points. In addition to points, the Hawks set a franchise record for total wins (52) and wins on the road (23). The Hawks led the league in shutouts (11) and shorthanded goals (13). Cristobal Huet and Antti Niemi provided solid goaltending. Duncan Keith finished second in team scoring with 69 points and was later awarded the Norris Trophy, just as I thought he would. Patrick Kane led the team with 88 points, ninth-best in the league.

I felt they were on the verge of winning the Cup if they had a little bit of luck and stayed healthy.

Many people will remember the overtime goal by Patrick Kane that won the Cup—and his wild celebration afterward, throwing his gloves up in the air—but I would go back to the shorthanded goal he scored in Game 5 of the first round against Nashville that was really important. Might be the biggest goal scored on this road to changing the recent history of the Hawks. The series was tied 2–2 and Nashville battled back from a 3–1 Hawks lead to go ahead 4–3 at 11:39 of the third period. With 1:03 left in the game, Marian Hossa was assessed a five-minute major for boarding. Joel Quenneville pulled Niemi for an extra attacker and after a terrible turnover by Martin Erat, Kane scored a shorthanded goal with 14 seconds left to tie the game. In overtime, Hossa came out of the penalty box and scored the game-winning goal at 4:07. That to me ignited the team going forward and the Hawks won the sixth game to win the series. They played Vancouver and beat the Canucks in six games to advance to the conference final. There they swept San Jose, which had the most points in the Western Conference in the regular season.

They faced Philadelphia in the Stanley Cup Final. I appeared on *Chicago Tonight* before the series with host Phil Ponce, who asked me if I thought the Hawks would win in four straight. I told him I expected it to go six or seven games but the Hawks would win. The Flyers finished with 88 points, 24 fewer than the Hawks, but they had faced some injuries and changed coaches. They beat the New York Rangers 2–1 in a shootout to qualify for the postseason on the final day of the regular season. But everything changes in the playoffs. The regular season goes out the window and a team can go on a roll. They were the seventh seed entering the playoffs and beat New Jersey in the first round of the playoffs, then defeated Boston in seven games after losing the first three and needing an overtime win in Game 4 to avoid being eliminated. The Flyers followed that up by downing Montreal. They were very similar in style to the Hawks. Before the series I thought it would be a high-scoring game because neither team had faced a team of this caliber.

Speaking of Philadelphia, I mentioned earlier that Bobby Clarke was one of my hockey idols. Another guy in the Flyers family who I think the world of is Paul Holmgren. When I played against him, I tried to stay the hell away from him. But off the ice, he's an awesome human. Holmer is respectful, a smart guy, and caring to his friends. I'm proud to call him one of mine.

The Hawks won the opener 6–5 and then the second game 2–1. Philadelphia refused to wilt and won the next two at home by scores of 4–3 in overtime and 5–3 in Game 4. The Hawks won the fifth game 7–4, setting up that historic sixth game that was punctuated by Kane's memorable goal.

There was some confusion after he scored it and I could not tell from our vantage point in the press box as the officials huddled to review the goal. But great goal-scorers know when the puck is in the net, so even though I lost sight of the puck, Kane knew the goal was going to count. All of his teammates followed suit in the wild celebration. There was hesitation on the bench by the Hawks coaches because they were still waiting for some sort of confirmation. A minute or so later, it was official.

The Stanley Cup drought finally ended, 49 years after the Hawks last won in 1961.

Knowing how hard it is to win the greatest trophy in the world, it is an amazing accomplishment. I played for the Hawks for five years and the closest I ever came to the Cup was my rookie year when we lost in the conference finals in six games to the Edmonton Oilers. I couldn't help but think what it would have been like if we had won the Cup then as a hometown guy.

CHAPTER 16

THE CALLS TO THE HALLS

I HAD SEEN SO MANY GUYS whose careers had started after mine who were inducted into the United States Hockey Hall of Fame that I wondered if I would ever be selected. That all changed in July 2012 when I received a call informing me I had been chosen for induction.

I had taken great pride in representing the U.S. in one Olympics, five World Championships, and three Canada Cups. I had a pretty good career in terms of points and games played, but suffice it to say it was very humbling to be selected for induction, especially to be included in the same year as Mike Modano and Mr. Lou Lamoriello.

I had never been to the induction ceremonies before. It is moved around to different cities each year and this one took place in Dallas, where Modo had the greatest year in his career. A massive American flag, draped on rigging behind the stage where the inductees sat, provided a spectacular background. There were about 300-400 people in the crowd. There were Hall of Fame dignitaries, former inductees, family and friends, former linemates at various stages of my career—including Pat LaFontaine and David A. Jensen from the Diaper Line—Dallas Stars owner Tom Hicks, and Murray Costello, a pioneer in Canadian hockey who was receiving the Wayne Gretzky International Award to honor international individuals who have made major contributions to the growth and advancement of ice hockey in the United States.

Diana and Eddie, Tommy, Alexandra, and Nicholas were there, along with my parents and Diana's parents, my brothers, and my nieces and nephews. My buddies Dom and Joe the Judge were there too. Modo, Mr. Lamoriello, and I were each told to limit our speeches to no more than 10 or 12 minutes, but as far as I was concerned, that wasn't happening. There were just too many people to highlight and mention because I wanted everyone in attendance to know everything I have in life was because of the great game of hockey. I was so grateful that so many people who had played a role in my life and career with there to help me celebrate this achievement. You see, it really wasn't about me; it was about all the people who had helped me along the way in this long, incredible journey.

DIANA OLCZYK
Eddie's mother
We were very humbled by Eddie's induction into the U.S. Hockey Hall of Fame. It was very nicely done and it was very overwhelming. It was another blessing we received. Being a mother, it brought tears for me, seeing your son there and receiving these accolades from people.

I looked upon this as a kid who was lucky enough to have achieved a dream and wanted people to know that hockey had been my life, both growing up under my parents' roof and being a parent myself. I noted the plaque we have in our home—WE INTERRUPT THIS FAMILY FOR HOCKEY—to provide an anecdote about how much the game has been part of the Olczyk family for two generations.

I had a speech prepared, but looking into the crowd there were so many things going through my mind and I wanted to make eye contact with the people I was referencing, in particular Diana and our children. In something as important as this, you want to share the emotion, the excitement, and the memory, and there's nothing better than doing that with the most important people in your life, starting with my parents, brothers, friends, and my wife and kids.

I wanted people to know my parents took me to and from games and practices and tournaments as a young kid who had fallen in love with hockey. They showed me how support starts at home, and that continues forward in my home. Life's too fast, and as I looked into the crowd at my parents, I thought of the unconditional love and support they showed for me and my brothers. And in a broader perspective, I wanted people to know my parents, my brothers, and my wife and kids have always been there for me for the wins and the losses, the good times and the bad.

RICKY OLCZYK
Eddie's brother

To be recognized for his achievements as a Hall of Famer was an incredible moment for our entire family. It was just a great couple of days. We were very honored and blessed that took place. So many things were going through our minds and in mine particularly, thinking of the sacrifices our parents made. They sacrificed not only financially but their time as well. How can you ever pay that back, someone's time, care, and love to help us along and to pursue and follow our dreams? That's what happened, and to cap that off with the U.S. Hockey Hall of Fame, that was just another fond, fond memory.

I congratulated Modo, with whom I had played many games for the U.S. in various competitions. He is someone I consider one of the greatest American-born players to play in the National Hockey League, and more than anything a friend. You know you have earned somebody's respect and trust when they call you asking for an opinion on a major decision, which was the case when Modo was thinking about signing with Detroit, the city in which he was born and raised, to play for the Red Wings. When you have earned the respect of a Mike Modano, you have truly arrived.

I also highlighted Mr. Lamoriello, who had become influential in my career beginning at the age of 16, when he was one of the coaches for Team USA who selected the players for the 1984 Olympic team. Mr. Lamoriello was coach of the East team, which had all of the youngest players. We have a relationship built on trust and respect, and I wanted to pay tribute to him for all he had done for U.S college hockey, USA Hockey, and the National Hockey League, in particular the New Jersey Devils, with whom he had won three Stanley Cups as a GM. Mr. Lamoriello has always had the time to say hello and always asks about my mom and dad, which is something that is very important to my family. I couldn't have been prouder to be inducted with him. He has always been a resource and an ally.

I also wanted to pay tribute to some of my linemates, beginning with Pat LaFontaine and David A. Jensen from the '84 Olympics. I joked that I was put on that line to slow it down a little bit. I also noted Troy and Curt, both of whom were in attendance, who were my linemates on the Clydesdales Line in Chicago. I also mentioned that I played on a line with Modo and Jeremy Roenick on Team USA, and on another line with Modo and Brett Hull. Brett, who was in the crowd, wore No. 16 on our U.S. teams and I wore No. 12. I joked that the goal-scorer got preference when choosing his number. And with no disrespect to all the lines I played on, I said this U.S. Hockey Hall of Fame line with Modo and Mr. Lamoriello would last forever.

I thanked Troy, Denis Savard, Darryl Sutter, and Ronnie Francis, who were teammates who showed me how to do things the right way and become a pro on and off the ice. I also thanked Bob Pulford and John Paddock, the two best coaches I ever played for and who understood my strengths and gave me opportunities.

I thanked the Chicago Blackhawks family, including the late Bill Wirtz and his sons, Peter and Rocky, and current executives John McDonough and Jay Blunk, all of whom played a role in my hockey journey.

And there were so many other people to thank: my former agents Rick Curran, Bill Watters, and Ronnie Salcer; former Meadowlands executive Hal Handel, for giving my start in broadcasting; USA Hockey executives Dave Fischer, Mark Tabrum, and Kevin McLaughlin; the many coaches I had growing up and in the Team USA program; the people who billeted me when I played Junior B in Stratford and during my year with the U.S. Olympic team; and the numerous trainers and equipment people who looked after me, some of whom still do.

I finished my speech by saying, "This honor has been and always will be tremendously tremendous."

If everything ended on the night I was inducted into the U.S. Hockey Hall of Fame, I don't know how anybody could not look back on my life and think it had not been pretty tremendous.

Collectively it was a great couple of days. Did I get emotional? Yeah. I fought off the tears pretty good, but I'm an emotional guy, always have been, always will be. It's one of the reasons Diana says she loves me. I'm sensitive. It's real. It's who I am. I don't know how to be any other way.

The following February, the Hawks made a special tribute to my Hall of Fame induction. When you get honored like that by your hometown team, it's very humbling. Like everything the Hawks do, it's more than first class. To think of me in that light and to recognize me after the Hall of Fame ceremonies was pretty awesome.

It began with the opening piano notes from the song "Hall of Fame" by The Script, featuring will.i.am. It was followed by an audio clip of me from my introductory press conference when I signed with the Hawks, when I said, "Being a Chicago guy, living and dying with the Blackhawks, this is truly an honor." Then came a video tribute on the giant scoreboard, photos of myself in youth hockey and the Olympics, and replays of some of my goals with the Hawks. For many of the goals I scored, they played the calls by Pat Foley, with him always calling me Eddie O. It concluded with my "tremendously tremendous" ending to my Hall of Fame speech.

I then walked on to the ice through a phalanx of young kids from the Niles youth hockey teams while arena announcer Harvey Wittenberg highlighted some of my achievements. I bowed a few times, pounded my heart, and waved to people in the crowd. Then I turned around and patted one of the young players on the head. Who knows, maybe there was a future Eddie Olczyk among those players. That was emotional, too, because it was almost like the show *This Is Your Life*. It was very cool.

JOHN McDONOUGH
Blackhawks president and CEO

Eddie symbolizes what it means to be a part of this franchise. He has a rich history and he's close with our fans. When you're going into the United States Hockey Hall of Fame, that's a major achievement and it has to be recognized here. And I wanted to be sure that we included his family. It was appropriately recognized and then some. We think he's an important part of our franchise.

The following May, I was inducted into the Chicagoland Sports Hall of Fame, honoring and memorializing athletes, coaches, teams, officials, media members, and others who have distinguished themselves with their contributions to sports. It started almost 25 years ago. The funny thing was this was the second time I'd been told I was being inducted. I had gotten the call once before, and I thought it was great, even more so when I was told it would take place in the Million Room on the clubhouse level of Hawthorne Racecourse. But when I was told the day of the event, I said I couldn't go because I had to work a preseason game for the Blackhawks. I was then told if I couldn't be there in person, I wouldn't be inducted. John McDonough thinks that's the funniest story. When they called this time, I was available.

I was inducted into the Italian American Sports Hall of Fame in September. Unfortunately, I was not able to be there for that one because I was working a Hawks game. My buddy Dominic Porro accepted it on my behalf. In 2004, I was inducted into the National Polish American Sports Hall of Fame. Being recognized with so many great athletes who have that heritage, I guess it means you've done something right and you are being recognized for it. Plus, it's your name and it's going to be around forever, especially with the Internet.

My folks are very proud of anything I do, regardless of whether it's publicly noted or not. I'm proud of them in turn and thank them for the love, support, and guidance they've given me over the years and to this day. Anything I have done is more than just an individual achievement; it's a family achievement.

CHAPTER 17

WITNESSING HISTORY

I HAD BEEN TO THE KENTUCKY DERBY once before as a fan in 2011 when Animal Kingdom won. I had the weekend off and NBC hooked me up with an all-access pass.

My second trip in 2015 turned out to be considerably more exciting because I was part of NBC's coverage of the race and the entire Triple Crown in what became horse racing history. How it all came about related to my handicapping and desire to be part of NBC's horse racing coverage.

While broadcasting the 2013 Stanley Cup playoffs, I gave out my Kentucky Derby picks. I liked Revolutionary, but I suggested using Orb and Golden Soul in exactas and trifectas. Orb won at almost 5½-1 odds, followed by Golden Soul at more than 34-1 and Revolutionary at more than 6-1. The $2 exacta paid $981.60 and the $1 trifecta $6,925.60. I also made a fractional wager, which allows bettors to use more horses in a bet at a fraction of the cost, on the superfecta bet for the top four finishers. The super paid $57,084 for a $2 ticket and I had bet it for 30 cents. Suffice it to say, I won a lot.

I was starting to feel pretty good about my handicapping and asked Sam Flood, the executive producer of NBC Sports, if there was any room for me on the Kentucky Derby broadcast. I had asked once a year for four or five years. When he started to see the successful results of my selections and people started talking about it, it gained some momentum.

Broadcaster Randy Moss, who is part of NBC Sports' coverage of the Triple Crown and also does some work for the Olympics, became a backer of mine. I met him in 2014 at the Winter Olympics where I was part of the hockey broadcast crew. Randy was at one of the games and I saw him and introduced myself to him between periods. We talked horse racing for the entirety of both intermissions. What a great chat.

Sam decided to give me a chance but I wouldn't be working the Triple Crown. On June 28, 2014, I debuted as part of NBC's broadcast of the Gold Cup from Santa Anita Racetrack in California. This was an audition and I could have easily picked the favorites, but that's not how I bet races and I had to be true to myself.

SAM FLOOD
NBC executive producer

Not only has he proven himself 100 percent as a handicapper, he's also proven himself as a broadcaster because he can ask the questions when he's doing interviews with people at the track. The respect that the people inside our broadcast who are pure horse racing people show for Eddie is through the roof.

The first race I did was the Senorita Stakes and I picked Sheza Smoke Show, trained by Peter Eurton, whose daughter, Britney, now works as part of NBC's horse racing coverage. Sheza Smoke Show had been off for three months, but I liked the fact jockey Joe Talamo was back aboard the filly and I thought she would do well off of the pace. It was a 10-horse field and the race unfolded just as I had predicted, and she split horse deep in the stretch and won at 10-1 odds.

The next race was the Gold Cup and it attracted a field of seven horses. I liked Majestic Harbor, who was about a 15-1 long shot in a field of only seven and won. Look, I got lucky and it all worked out. Sam was very excited afterward but I said, "If I can bat .300 the whole year with my picks I'd be more than happy. This ain't going to happen very often." But it felt great. I knew I could do it, I just needed for Sam to give me the chance. I promised myself I would not let him down.

MIKE "DOC" EMRICK
NBC broadcaster

Eddie didn't push Sam, but it was pretty obvious when he got the first four horses right in the 2014 Derby that by the time I got to the airport I was telling everyone in our crew we've got to show that video next week. We ran it the next week.

One of our cameramen put down $100 and picked the first four horses like Eddie did and made $10,000. Cameramen aren't paid a lot of money. They are paid okay, but aren't living on the Riviera. The cameraman came to me and said, "I made a ton of money off of Eddie's picks. What kind of liquor does he like? I'll get him a big bottle of whatever he likes." I said, "You've got the wrong guy there because he doesn't drink, but he likes desserts and he likes ice cream, so why don't you get him a gift card." I don't know what the cameraman did, but he wanted to do something for Eddie because he had turned $100 into $10,000.

I did a few more races that year and Sam told me I'd be part of the 2015 Triple Crown coverage, which includes the Kentucky Derby, Preakness Stakes, and Belmont Stakes. I'd been watching the Triple Crown my whole life, and now I was going to get this chance to be on center stage. Amazing.

Being at Churchill Downs four years later as part of NBC's broadcast, I still looked at it as a fan. I would have felt differently if I hadn't been to the Derby before—it would have been much more intimidating—but I felt like I had arrived after my work at the Meadowlands in 2004 and continuing through to my more recent work starting with the Gold Cup card.

It was noted on the broadcast I'd had success with some of my picks, including winning $500,000 in a Pick 6 betting only $168, and that I knew my way around the track. But in the beginning, there was always that feeling among some people that I was a hockey guy doing horse racing. Today, there are people who come up to me and say, "Hey, you're the horse racing guy who does hockey," which is a great compliment.

Even though I had a big maiden voyage at Santa Anita with Sheza Smoke Show and Majestic Harbor, 99.9 percent of the people watching the Derby had no clue about that. They could have just introduced me as a handicapper, but it was a great cross promotion for horse racing and hockey and NBC really embraced that, which was great because both of those are among major properties for the network, along with golf and soccer.

Bob Neumeier, who had been part of the coverage for a long time, was the other handicapper, and I loved working with him. He was a hockey guy, having broadcast Boston Bruins and Hartford Whalers games, and I became close with him and his wife, Michelle, both salt of the earth people. Neumy is a gregarious guy and a wonderful storyteller, and I'll get to one in a bit. Some of the horsemen knew me because I had been part of NBC's horse racing coverage and I had gotten to know a lot of the jockeys over the years. Gradually the horsemen came to know me as Eddie Olczyk, the horse racing handicapper and not Eddie Olczyk, the former hockey player. I'll always remember crossing paths at Belmont Park in New York in 2018 with Hall of Famer Shug McGaughey and reintroducing myself. We had met once before when I was with the Rangers, and this time I wished him good luck in the Belmont Stakes and he said, "Thanks, Eddie." I couldn't believe Shug McGaughey knew me, which was really cool.

For the 2015 Derby, I liked Dortmund, which came into the race undefeated in six starts, including the Santa Anita Derby in its last outing. The horse was the second choice in the field at more than 4-1, which was good value. The favorite was American Pharoah, a winner of four consecutive races, including the Arkansas Derby in his last start, at just under 3-1. Dortmund seized the lead fairly early into the race and led all the way to the top of the stretch and then faded, finishing third, more than 3 lengths back of American Pharoah.

Did I feel like I had blown my big chance? No, that's horse racing. Any horseplayer will tell you after the race, "How did I not have this horse?"

I liked American Pharoah for the Preakness Stakes two weeks later in Baltimore at Pimlico Racecourse. The race was run in a rainstorm and the track was sloppy. It was dangerous out there. As I walked across the track before the race I was thinking, this is crazy. But American Pharoah, who was the heavy favorite at just under even money, led from the start and won by 7 lengths. He came into the Belmont Stakes three weeks later trying to sweep the Triple Crown. It had not happened since Affirmed in 1978, and there had been 13 horses since that time that came into the Belmont looking to make history and failed, the last being California Chrome the year before. My feeling was no one was going to beat American Pharoah.

But here's my Neumy story, and I'll preface it by saying he loved to have fun and bust my balls every once in a while, whether we were on camera or not. In the Acorn Stakes, a Grade 1 race on the undercard of Belmont Stakes day, I had just gone on our NBC broadcast and picked a horse, By the Moon, that was 30-1, the second-longest shot on the betting board in the field of 12 fillies. Jockey Jose Ortiz was aboard and he had her behind the speed early in the race and took the lead turning for home. She had a 2-length lead at the top of the stretch and Ortiz had her in the four path, meaning he was closer to the middle of the track than the rail. On this day, the rail was not the place to be because it was deeper than the middle. For the horses running closer to the rail, it was like running uphill. For the horses closer to the middle, it was like they were running downhill. Track conditions change for a variety of reasons, sometimes during the course of a card. Sometimes the rail is the best place to be, sometimes it is the worst. Smart handicappers note the track bias. Ortiz was guiding her closer to the rail and here comes jockey John Velasquez aboard Curalina, a 7-1 shot trained by Todd Pletcher. The horse had a brutal start at the gate but was making up ground and came roaring down the center of the track and nipped By the Moon by a neck at the wire. I would have made a huge score if Ortiz kept her in the middle of track. She wins 100 percent, I have no doubt in my mind. I had the winners in the last two races and was alive in the Pick 3, the daily double, and wins and place bets. Honestly, it cost me at least $100,000.

We came back on camera about 45 mins after that tough beat and Neumy starts our segment saying, "I have always loved Eddie Olczyk—a hockey guy, a Brother Rice High School guy, a handicapper—but I really love how he just put $700 of losing tickets into his satchel."

"Way to sell me down the river Neumy after that tough beat," I said. (Hey Neumy, full disclosure: those tickets were worth a tad more than $700.)

The great chemistry with Neumy was the same as with Mike Lange, Doc Emrick, and Pat Foley. Neumy taught me a lot right away about so many things and I'll be forever grateful for that. I learned a long time ago sometimes it's better to just keep your mouth shut and your ears and your eyes open.

American Pharoah was bet down to 75 cents on the dollar, even lower odds than the Preakness. Once again, he dominated the race from the start and won by 5½ lengths. Simply as a fan it was the greatest sporting event I was a part of because history had been made. The reaction of all the people in the crowd at Belmont Park was incredible, one of those things where you had to be there to appreciate it.

What a way to come on to the scene as a rookie broadcaster in the Triple Crown. The winning trainer was Bob Baffert, whom I have become close with over the years along with his wife, Jill, and their son Bode. I first met Bob as a fan in California when he was just starting off as a thoroughbred trainer in the early '90s and I was with trainer Tom Proctor. I met Bob again at the 2010 Olympics in Vancouver when I was coming out of the elevator of the Pan Pacific Hotel. I introduced myself and said I was a former National Hockey League player and was in Vancouver working for NBC as part of its men's hockey coverage and that we had met once before. Bob was either preoccupied or it didn't resonate with him or he didn't care. It was definitely one of the three, but knowing him now as I do and having become good friends with him, I'd like to think he was preoccupied.

BOB BAFFERT
Thoroughbred horse trainer
He loves the horses. He follows horse racing and he's part of the racing community. You can tell when he speaks, he believes in what he is saying. He's a student of the sport and he's learning and he's not afraid to ask questions. He puts his money where his mouth is and that's a big difference. Horse racing is fun and it's really exciting, but he makes it more exciting. You can tell it's not a job to him. He really enjoys it. He loves it.

* * *

I had to refocus on hockey after the Triple Crown. The Hawks had just split the first two games of the Stanley Cup Final against the Tampa Bay Lightning. They split the next two games, and then Chicago won the next two, capturing the Cup at the United Center, nine days after Pharoah's historic win. It was the Hawks' third Cup since 2010.

It was a trying time, physically, mentally, and emotionally, although the extra week in between the Preakness Stakes and the Belmont Stakes helped. But what an experience!

In the 2016 Kentucky Derby, the horse that everyone was talking about was Nyquist, named after Detroit Red Wings player Gustav Nyquist. The owner, Paul Reddam, was a hockey fan who lived in Windsor, Ontario, on the Canadian side of the border opposite Detroit. Mr. Reddam, trainer Doug O'Neill, and jockey Mario Gutierrez collectively won the Derby in 2012 with I'll Have Another, which went on to win the Preakness. But I'll Have Another's chance at making history ended when he had to be scratched the day before the Belmont Stakes because of an ankle injury. Nyquist was the favorite at just under 5-2 odds and I gave out the exactor with Exaggerator at just over 5-1. It paid $30.60. And as I often say, sometimes you have to take what the track gives you. Exaggerator won the Preakness with Nyquist finishing third by almost 4 lengths, so right away the Triple Crown vibe was much different.

In 2017, Always Dreaming, the Derby favorite at just under 5-1, won and once again there was a hockey angle. One of the owners of the horse was Vinnie Viola, owner of the Florida Panthers. Always Dreaming finished eighth of 10 starters in the Preakness, so again the possibility of a Triple Crown sweep was immediately over.

Sometimes it seems like there isn't enough time in the day to prepare for the playoff games and get ready for the Triple Crown races. We do two days of horse racing, including the card the day before, and the prep on that is pretty intense. What has happened lately is I have been taken off of hockey coverage from the early part of the week until after the horse races, and then back to hockey. Previous to that I was doing a game on a Tuesday night, traveling to the city where the Triple Crown race was taking place and getting ready for the two horse racing shows, which is four hours on Friday and seven hours on Saturday. I told Sam and producer Rob Hyland it would be great if I could have an extra day off and both were okay with that.

But all of that was a cakewalk compared to what I was about to face: chemotherapy and battling cancer.

CHAPTER 18

GOING 12 ROUNDS WITH CANCER

IN MID-AUGUST, A FEW WEEKS after I underwent the surgery that removed the tumor, Diana and I traveled to Northwestern Hospital to meet with oncologist Dr. Mary Mulcahy. She was going to explain what would transpire with the treatments, what medicines I would receive, the side effects, the schedule, and the overall routine.

The meeting lasted exactly 47 minutes. I know that because I looked at the clock when the meeting began and again when it ended. During the entire time I had a thousand-yard stare. Basically, it was a conversation between Diana and Dr. Mulcahy. I was listening but nothing was registering. I was having an out-of-body experience. Am I really here? Is this really happening to me? I'm in an oncologist's office and I'm going to start cancer treatments and I have to come here every two weeks for the next six months? How am I going to do that?

The only thing I remember hearing from Dr. Mulcahy was, "Eddie, look at me. I'm here to cure you, not treat you. Do you understand the difference?"

We scheduled the first treatment for Monday, September 11, starting at 7:15 AM. That would be the schedule for 12 treatments, every two weeks. Diana and I left at about 5:45, traveling to the same hospital I had been transported to in an ambulance for the surgery. I had a nauseous feeling on the way there, not knowing what I would feel like when the chemo hit me for the first time.

When we arrived, there were other cancer patients, some of whom had been there numerous times before. As I would learn, we were all there for the same reason, even if we all had a different story and dosages. The treatment began with taking blood work to make sure my hemoglobin level, which indicates iron deficiency, was at a certain level. I was then hooked up to an IV drip and given anti-nausea medicine, vitamins, and steroids to provide energy, because the chemo knocks you out. If you did straight chemo for two weeks, you'd be on your back the whole time. I took one type of chemo at the hospital and when that ended they hooked me up with round two of a different type of chemo to go home with. After that, I began the chemo and I immediately became aware of the rhythm of it, which had a puffing sound similar to an air gun going off every 90 seconds. I began to feel sick and started vomiting and that's when it hit me that this was real. Hospitals have a certain smell to begin with, and once you start receiving chemo, you reek of it.

I returned home and continued the treatment with a fanny pack and a pump with a port connected to my chest. The nurse came to my home and unhooked me two days later. After the first treatment, I started a calendar to mark off the dates to my final treatment. I needed something to envision my goal. On the calendar, I set milestones for myself to help pass the time.

Get back in the booth for hockey and horse racing, in particular the Breeders' Cup World Thoroughbred Championships in early November.

Thanksgiving.

My daughter's graduation from the University of Alabama.

Christmas.

Super Bowl Sunday.

As an athlete, I was goal-oriented and controlled what I could on a day-to-day basis. I took the same approach dealing with my cancer battle.

I lived in the basement because I did not want to be in any normal surroundings. I just wanted to go down there and be by myself in the quietest place in the house. Diana would bring me food and just the smell of it would make me throw up. Macaroni and cheese would really make me sick. I used to love macaroni and cheese but I haven't had it since.

We got used to the routine. We'd get home from the hospital at 1:30 in the afternoon, and I'd go down to the basement and be there until 7:00 or 8:00. I'd come upstairs and see Diana and the dogs—Lily and Daisy—and then would go downstairs again. My sleeping patterns were terrible. I'd fall asleep and wake up at 4:00 in the morning. Then you hear the machine go off and you're looking at the clock and you want to fast forward the world.

Pretty soon, the side effects had worn me down. I was vomiting badly, had no control of my bowels, bad nose bleeds, headaches, and neuropathy, which is coldness in the nerve endings in the fingers and feet that made it hard to button a shirt and pull up a zipper. It was just terrible. How was I going to make it to the final treatment on February 21? I had basically had enough and wanted to pull the port out of my chest and quit. How can I or anyone else who is battling live like this? I was a beaten human not even two weeks into this six-month battle. Diana grabbed me and said, "Fight for me, fight for our kids, and fight for the people who love you."

I was crying because I was in tremendous pain and couldn't control anything. I just didn't feel human, but Diana basically got me on the straight and narrow. I took a deep breath and decided to take it one treatment at a time. I'd wait for Wednesday when my nurse Joe would unhook me and then I'd start over again two weeks later.

DIANA OLCZYK
Eddie's wife

I think going through chemo treatment and just seeing how it affected him physically and mentally, you need someone to give you a shake. I think all of us every now and then fall into a dark place where you go, woe is me, but you've got to find the fight. I was like, "We're going through it this way. You've got to fight for me, for the kids, for the many people who love you and are counting on you. If you don't have the ability right now to do this for yourself, look around you and do it for us."

There were many Mondays Diana and I were emotionally drained just sitting in the waiting room before going in for treatment. Being a public figure, especially in Chicago, a lot of people recognized me and came up to me to tell their stories. Some of them were absolutely heartbreaking. They took their treatments and lived day-to-day because they didn't want to know the prognosis. We felt for them and it became hard not to get emotional. It really gave me insight into cancer and the battles people go through, and their bravery. I saw courage every time I went to the hospital on those Mondays.

I started receiving calls and texts from well-wishers and I was surprised because many were people I didn't know that well. One of them left me a 30-second phone message. I'm not sure how this person got my number, but it was so nice to hear words of encouragement from someone I didn't even know. A lot of people sent me cards through NBC or the Blackhawks. I got a couple of hundred pieces of mail a week.

On September 29, with the NHL season about to begin, my Blackhawks broadcast partner, Pat Foley, threw out the first pitch at a Cubs game at Wrigley Field and later sang "Take Me Out to the Ball Game" during the seventh-inning stretch. He wore a Cubs jersey which had OLCZYK 16 on the back. He reversed it so everyone could see my name, and before he began to sing he said, "Let Eddie O. hear you all the way to the suburbs."

I had no idea he was planning to do any of this. I just happened to be watching the game at home with Diana because I'm such a huge Cubs fan and watch as much as I can. It was so awesome that he would think of me and want everybody to think of me. It really meant a lot. I thought, is this what it will look and feel like when I am not alive? I know he was doing it in my honor and my memory, but Diana and I were crying. I texted Pat shortly after thanking him for that unbelievable gesture. Cubs TV play-by-play man Len Kasper sent me a text, too, wishing me well. It was an emotional, inspiring day like no other.

Around this time, I received a package from Hall of Fame thoroughbred trainer Bob Baffert, with whom I had developed an incredible relationship as part of NBC's coverage of racing. The package contained a shoe worn by Arrogate prior to the running of the Dubai World Cup on March 25. It also included a message that said, "We all know how that started and how he finished." The Dubai World Cup is one of the biggest and richest races in the world with a $10 million purse. Arrogate had won the 2016 Horse of the Year honors and rather than retire him immediately to stud, the decision was made to train him for the Dubai race and then send him to stud. Arrogate had a poor beginning in the race and was last in the field of 14. Turning for home, he was 8 lengths back of the lead and running widest of all. Then Arrogate turned it on and with about 300 yards to the wire he seized the lead. It was a brilliant end for an incredible horse. So Bob was pretty much saying I was down but not out and I would recover just like Arrogate. That's how I took it. The package also contained a beautiful note from Bob's son Bode. Bob's wife, Jill, wrote a nice card and Bob signed it.

Arrogate is the best horse I have ever seen in person, better than American Pharoah, Justify, or Cigar. To get something like that from Bob and his family, it brightened my day. I put the horseshoe up on the wall in my office. I thanked him right away and told him it was totally unnecessary but that it meant a lot to me that he took the time to do that. It was just another example of how communicating to someone who is going through this type of battle can mean so much. In my case, I was beginning to feel like I had a team of thousands of people rooting for me and I didn't want to let anybody down. This package was another thing to keep me battling.

Bob suffered a heart attack in 2012 in his hotel room while in Dubai for the Dubai World Cup. He recovered and admitted it changed his life. In the context of what happened to him and what I was going through, the horseshoe meant so much for so many different reasons. It was nice when he called and said, "How's it going, Champ?"

BOB BAFFERT
Thoroughbred horse trainer

He's always been great to me and my wife and my kids. We just wanted to pick his spirits up. I was hoping that shoe would bring him some luck. He was depressed. When I had my health scare, I thought I was toast. I didn't realize how many people were worried about me, and that made me feel good. When he came back to the Triple Crown, everybody was just thrilled to see him. Eddie O. is like part of the team and everybody was excited to see him again.

On October 7, I attended the Blackhawks game against the Columbus Blue Jackets to do a first-period interview with Pat. It was my first time out publicly and I wanted to talk about my cancer and just lay what was happening out for people. The Hawks showed an image of me on the giant scoreboard while I was sitting in the Blackhawks suite for the game and the crowd went wild, giving me a standing ovation and shouting, "Edd-ie, Edd-ie, Edd-ie." Pat said it was like I was back playing with the

Hawks wearing my No. 16 jersey. I was touched by the reaction. The players on both benches stood and acknowledged me and the coaches were clapping. I felt everybody was with me. My attitude all along was this was a team effort, and to get that type of reception made me feel really good. I felt right at home.

JAY BLUNK
Blackhawks executive vice president

John and I wanted him to know that we were in full support of whatever was best for him. As the treatments for his cancer progressed, Eddie had a change of heart and told us that the quiet time away from the game was actually not good after all. He asked if he could come back between his treatments. The entire organization was elated at first, but worried about Eddie's long-term health. However, you could feel his enthusiasm through the phone. Eddie's willingness to allow us to go on the journey with him enabled many of us to feel comfortable with asking him the tough questions. Many times, his voice would waver. My voice would waver. But we both ended the conversation with something constructive...every time. Eddie's body was fighting with everything he had. We were all in the fight together.

Pat and I had not discussed what he would ask me and it turned out to be emotional, funny, and generally provided me with something I needed. Pat began the interview saying every off-season, fans would ask us how the Blackhawks were going to do, but this time the first question people asked him was about me. I took a deep breath and said, "We're in a battle right now and we're going through our treatments." I acknowledged the support I had from Pat; the Blackhawks organization, including owner Rocky Wirtz, president John McDonough, and executive vice president Jay Blunk; team doctor Dr. Michael Terry, who had spearheaded everything with me with through all my treatments; and the great people at Northwestern Hospital. I also acknowledged my family and friends, all the Blackhawk fans, the hockey fans, the horse racing fans, Hawks players, and coach Joel Quenneville and his staff. And I thanked all the people who sent me cards and texts and emails.

I told Pat I had good days and bad days in my battle, but that this was a good week. I appreciated the opportunity to come to the United Center and see a lot of familiar faces. I talked about how my mom and dad, my brothers, Diana, and my kids were all in this battle together. When I talked about the support of Diana, I became really emotional and had to fight back the tears.

"I'm a lucky guy," I said. "She is the straw that stirs the drink."

Then I told Pat that Diana made him a batch of cookies and Pat howled.

"I've always loved her and I love her more," he said. "Buddy, everybody loves you."

I also talked about the Columbus Blue Jackets, a team that had reached out many a night to see how I was feeling, with a special thanks to team president John Davidson, head coach John Tortorella, TV play-by-play man Jeff Rimer, and TV analyst Billy Davidge (a cancer battler as well). The Jackets went way beyond the call of duty. Pat and I do shoutouts during our broadcasts and we knew how important it is to the people we're reaching out to, but when the skate is on the other foot, it really hits home. I said I was overwhelmed with the support and hoped to be back sooner rather than later.

"I'm just going day-to-day, partner," I said to Pat. "Your incredible support, the texts, the visits, the phone calls, I love you and I feel like we're going through this together. I'm going to beat this thing."

I then mentioned how someone once asked me, if I got in a wrestling match with a gorilla or a grizzly bear, would I stop when they're tired or when I was tired? I replied that obviously I'm going to stop when *they* are tired. I wasn't going to stop fighting this cancer until I got that clean bill of health.

Pat said it was great that so many people had reached out to me offering support and added, "This is really good juju. You've done so many things for so many people, partner, now it's time for a little getback. I know there's been plenty of days when you need a little boost and a little energy and a little assistance and we're all here to give it to you. Even people who don't know you want you to know how much they are thinking about you and are praying for you and that never hurts."

I reiterated that it had been absolutely overwhelming and again thanked Dr. Terry, Dr. Ruchim, Dr. Strong, Dr. Mulcahy, my infusion nurse Miss Caroline, and all the people who were on my team. I told Pat I wanted to get back as soon as I could to the broadcast booth with him.

Pat put an arm around me and I said, "I'm looking forward to getting my crayons and doing a little teaching."

Pat let out a huge "Yes!"

"It's great to be back and I feel like I'm at home and I'll be forever thankful," I said. "I don't think I'll have enough time on this earth to thank everybody, but hopefully everybody knows how important it's been to me and my family. Forever is a long time, but I'll be thanking people forever."

I told him when I beat cancer I planned to help other cancer patients along the way and noted all the stories I had heard from fellow patients and how I wanted to be there for them.

He told me he loved having me beside him in the announcer's booth again and gave me a huge hug and told me I'd be back sooner rather than later.

* * *

A few days later I began my third treatment and soon after developed a blood clot that made me feel like my right leg was disintegrating. I was at home and could not put any weight on it. We were having our patio deck redone and the gentleman who was doing it, Bryan Hand, a firefighter by day, drove me to the emergency room of Lake Forest Hospital. Diana eventually met me there.

Before the fifth game of the National League Championship Series at Wrigley Field, the Hawks tweeted a message of encouragement to the Cubs on my behalf. The Cubs were down three games to one to the Los Angeles Dodgers. My message was, "It's not how many times you get knocked down, it's how many times you get up." The Cubs posted that on the scoreboard before the first pitch. Unfortunately, the Cubs lost the game 11–1 and were eliminated. I guess my tweet came up empty.

I started to do media interviews because there were so many requests, which surprised me because I wasn't aware I was that important. Some of the requests came in through the Blackhawks, others from NBC, and they weren't just from sports outlets; they were also from news channels. They all wanted to hear my story and I started to think that by doing interviews maybe I could help somebody. Immediately I had people contact me to say thanks for sharing my story because either they or a family member had gone through the same thing. Instead of just writing them back, I'd call them. I was relatable to these people because I was living the same life. What I was sharing and going through was exactly what they were experiencing, so they felt connected.

I had one young boy ask if I could talk to his friend who was going through chemo treatments. I was given the phone number to his hospital room and he was aware I would be calling. His mother answered the phone and she said he wasn't available, so I said, "Could you please tell him that Eddie Olczyk of the Blackhawks called?"

I could tell she didn't know who I was, so I gave her my number and the boy called me back. He said, "My mom is the only person in the world who doesn't know you are." I told him that was okay.

I felt it was important to help and be a leader when it came to dealing with these battles. Tony Cachey, a former teammate of mine at Brother Rice High School, had developed colon cancer almost four months after

I was diagnosed. He's a big coach in the community in girls' hockey, so I texted him and tried to help him through his fight.

I had an open invitation from both the Blackhawks and NBC to come back to work. John McDonough essentially said if I felt like working, I could, even if was just for an hour before a game. Sam Flood said the same thing—that there was no pressure. If I wanted to do one game a month, I could do that. If I felt well enough to do more than that, I could do that, too. I hope all bosses will be that understanding to their employees as John and Sam were for me because it meant a lot to have that support.

SAM FLOOD
NBC executive producer

I was one of the first people he called after he learned he had cancer. I'm a survivor of prostate cancer. I had to leave the Stanley Cup Final after the sixth game in 2009 to go for surgery the following day and basically told no one outside of my family until that moment.

I had visited him after his second chemo because I knew he was struggling. He was in and out of it, and there were periods when he just sat there in tremendous pain and couldn't talk. You could see it was just tearing him apart. At the end I said, "Eddie, if you feel better, I want to roll a live truck here and want you to talk to the NBC team." Eddie and I mapped it out and he thought he would be okay because it would be in the right cycle for the chemo.

All the talent was there, probably about 60 people, and we went through our plans for the season. It was the first time Eddie wasn't there. I told the group Mike Milbury was going to be in Eddie's slot and then I said, "I have a guy who can give Mike Milbury some advice on how to count too many men on the ice. Edzo?" Eddie popped up via a two-way feed and it was the most powerful 10 minutes with everyone cheering and celebrating that Eddie was there.

By this time, I had come to understand the chemo treatment and the immediate side effects. Treatment Monday; unhooked Wednesday; recover Thursday, Friday, and Saturday; and start feeling a little bit better on Sunday. Maybe I could start working on my off weeks.

I felt well enough to do my first game for NBCSN on October 18 and texted Sam Flood, who said, "The seat is yours." The Hawks were playing in St. Louis in the Wednesday Rivalry Game. That morning I went to the arena to talk to the Hawks players. In an interview with *USA Today*'s Kevin Allen, Sam said what I was doing is a key to normalcy because there is nothing normal about fighting cancer. He said what was normal for me is the Wednesday Night Rivalry game, being at the rink, and being around people, the Blackhawks, the Blues, and Doc Emrick. He thought the rink is a special outlet for me.

I told Tracey Meyers, who was working for NBC Sports Chicago and now works for NHL.com, that it felt normal and comfortable to be back. I felt invigorated seeing a lot of familiar faces, "guys busting my chops and getting a lot of well-wishes." She interviewed Hawks forward Ryan Hartman, who said, "I was pretty excited to see him back. It's definitely a presence you know when you're watching games, that voice you heard growing up. He looks good, looks healthy. He's in a battle but he looks really good."

Joel Quenneville added, "We think about him every day and we've had the pleasure of having him come by a couple of times. Having him here today for a road game is great to know, but he has a tough battle ahead of him and he's doing everything he can to fight it. We support him every single day."

I told Tracey I was overwhelmed by everybody's well-wishes and said it was the best medicine I'd had in a long time.

The Blues recognized me as well that night. What a great reception from those fans and players. Thanks to Blues chairman Tom Stillman, GM Doug Armstrong, and their entire organization for that gesture.

It was great to be beside Doc for the game. We did an interview and I talked about how cancer had become the latest challenge in my life. I added that I wanted to be on *The Today Show* and that Smucker's jar with Al Roker and Dylan Dreyer.

The next night in Chicago, I did my first local game with the Hawks. The Hawks lost to the Oilers 2–1 in overtime, but it was great to be back.

I really wanted to enjoy Thanksgiving, so I took a break from the chemo routine with Dr. Mulcahy's approval. I was almost at the halfway point of the 12 treatments. Once I got to that point it was like I was halfway home. That was one of the goals I set for myself. By that point, the worst part of it had ended and now it was just following it through to the end.

A few days later I attended the Blackhawks game against the Anaheim Ducks and dropped the ceremonial opening puck with nine-year-old cancer patient Lauren Graver of Mount Prospect. We were there to participate in the Hawks' Hockey Fights Cancer, a National Hockey League initiative. Every year the local Make-A-Wish Foundation chooses a young cancer patient to be an ambassador for Hockey Fights Cancer and to raise awareness about pediatric cancer. Lauren, a fourth-grade student at Lions Park School, had a rare muscle-based cancer called rhabdomyosarcoma. About 10 days before the Hawks asked me to be part of this, I was supposed to start my fourth treatment and I knew how bad I would feel afterward. So, we delayed the treatment by a few hours at Northwestern so I could go directly to the United Center.

If you look at video of the puck drop, I was holding on tightly to Lauren. I think I was more nervous than she was. After the puck drop, I drove to the south side of Chicago to attend a wake for Frank DiCristina Sr.—Mr. D., as I called him—who owned the rink where I skated much of my whole life. It was one of the most emotional and unique days I experienced during my treatments, paying my respect to his son, Frankie Jr. This was a few weeks after another friend, Rick Faron, had passed away after battling kidney issues for years. The hockey world also lost broadcaster Dave Strader to bile duct cancer. Dave had been the voice of the Phoenix Coyotes and also did NHL games and the Olympics for NBC. We had worked together on the second NHL Outdoor Classic in 2009, when he subbed for Doc, who had laryngitis. Overall, it was not a good feeling with all these people dying while I was battling cancer. It was a real struggle to get through that period mentally.

JOHN McDONOUGH
Blackhawks president and CEO
I know that Lauren and the Graver family felt very supported that the NHL has the Hockey Fights Cancer initiative, and Eddie had someone he connected with who was going through this. I felt as if he really helped her through very difficult times.

I did an interview around this time with my good friend, broadcaster David Kaplan, on his ESPN 1000 radio show, *Kap & Co.*, in Chicago. Kap and I either talk or text every day. The first day I was in the hospital, Kap tried to contact me several times, but I wasn't feeling well enough to respond. I called him Sunday morning and told him we had a big problem and asked him to come down to Northwestern Hospital. When he got there, I was crying and told him the doctors thought I had colon cancer. Henceforth, he increased the number of times we dialoged in a day. From the start of my chemotherapy, it was like 10 times a day between talking on the phone, texting, and visiting me, anything to help get my mind off what I was going through.

He asked me if he could do a TV interview with me once I went public with the news. I wasn't sure if I could emotionally hold it together, but once I was feeling up to it, I agreed. I talked in the interview about the dates and goals that I set. Kap said he always thought of me as invincible, that nothing could stop me. He asked me if it was okay to be scared and I took a deep breath. He wasn't just asking about being scared for myself, but for Diana, our kids, my friends, and my fans. It hit a nerve and I began to cry.

"Sometimes I feel like I'm letting my family down and my friends down and I don't like to see people hurt," I said.

Diana had been with me through every step of this and I recalled the wedding vows we took 29 years earlier, notably the words "in sickness and in health." Kap asked me what it was like at home with me and Diana and the dogs on a random day. I told him that the dogs instinctively knew when I came home that something was wrong and put their chins on my legs and just sat with me. That was comforting and great medicine. I told him on the days that I'm not doing treatments I laugh and I cry and get mad at him when I listen to his radio show.

That's the kind of relationship and friendship I have with Kap. I could say something like that when moments before I was crying. I told him sometimes I had to call in to the show to set him straight because I'm pretty much the only one who will. He's an easy target for me; his producers Danny Zederman and Chris Bleck keep him honest for me in the studio. Listening to the show helped pass the time.

Kap talked about how it seems that while I may be the big, tough hockey player and voice of the Blackhawks and NHL, Diana is the rock. I acknowledged she is tough.

"Unlike you, I'm not embarrassed to say she is in charge around here. I got lucky," I said.

The interview ended with a shot of me giving a thumbs-up to the fans during one of the games I broadcasted.

Kap says it was the hardest interview he's ever done in his 32-year career because we have a connection unlike any other he's ever had. He was trying not to cry because he didn't want it to be about him. It was really hard for him when I talked about how Diana and I wanted to be at Eddie's wedding. He is super close with our kids and as I talked about it, he says he was praying that I would live to see that day.

* * *

In early November, the Breeders' Cup World Championships took place at Del Mar in California. This was one of the dates I had penciled in on my calendar. It took place over two days and totaled 14 races.

I gave out my picks on Xpressbet.com, with which I am affiliated. For the Classic, the last and biggest race, I picked Gun Runner to win and Collected to place second. The focus was on Arrogate, the horse I'd picked several times in major races and the favorite to win the Classic. I noted in my Xpressbet analysis of the race that if the race was held anywhere but Del Mar, he'd be my choice, but he didn't handle the track as well as other tracks. I liked Gun Runner because he was on a roll and had a huge tactical edge because he could go to the lead or sit just off it. I also thought jockey Florent Geroux knew exactly which buttons to push with the horse. Gun Runner could handle the distance of a mile and a quarter, which would be farther than he'd ever gone. I liked Collected to finish second because I thought he could get loose on the lead and the contour of the track would play to his running style, combined with already having a massive race at Del Mar at the race distance. I also said he was going to be tough to pass. I also did a two-way with Bob Costas from my basement and he asked me how I was feeling and how I saw the Classic unfolding.

The race unfolded just as I predicted. Gun Runner led from start to finish and won easily, followed by Collected, which ran in second the whole trip. Arrogate, the race favorite, ran fifth. Gun Runner paid $6.80 to win and the exacta with Collected paid $17. It felt great to be right and to cash as well.

There was another interesting sidebar to the win. In the summer, I made a $500 bet with Kap on his radio show: he said the Chicago Cubs were going to win 94 games and I said they wouldn't. The Cubs exceeded 94 wins and I owed him $500. I went to get my hair cut one day and I looked at a pamphlet for the Ross K. MacNeill Foundation for Pediatric Cancer. The foundation was started in memory of Ross, an 11-year-old who played hockey. He passed away in 2013 after a four-year battle with brain cancer. The pamphlet indicated the foundation was doing a fundraiser to raise awareness of pediatric cancer.

A couple of days later I was on the radio and Kap asked, "You got my $500?"

I said I did but was going to add $250 to it and bet all of it on the Breeders' Cup Classic and donate the money we win to the Ross MacNeill Foundation. Kap was all for it.

We had listeners calling in making donations. Some of our colleagues at the station chipped in with $50 or $100 and we received donations from Dino's Sports Fan Shop and Rich Friedman from Home Court Advantage. It added up to $1,700. We guaranteed we'd give $750 to the foundation no matter what happened.

I bet $750 on Gun Runner to win and did a $400 exacta box with Gun Runner and Collected, so they had to finish in the top two in either order. I bet the rest of trifectas. When Gun Runner won and the exacta box hit, we won $7,640 for the charity. The station had one of those oversized checks and presented it to Ross' mother, Kim, who came into the studio. A $500 bet on the Cubs turned into $7,640 for the charity. I think it was meant to be. That was a lot of fun.

* * *

Alexandra graduated from the University of Alabama in December. One of my goals had been to be there to see it. Diana and I attended the ceremony and Diana took a photo of Zandra and me that my daughter posted on her Instagram account with the caption, "Words wouldn't do my thoughts justice on how proud I am of my dad. All the strength that was shown through these months just goes to show who he really is. You showed so many how brave you are & that a fighter, not just on the ice, can beat cancer. All of this just goes to show that nothing is impossible & I'm so blessed to say you just proved that."

All of the kids came home for Christmas, which was great. Eddie had been at Bemidji State in Minnesota working as the assistant coach of the hockey team. Tommy was in Indianapolis playing for the Indy Fuel of the East Coast Hockey League. Nicky had come home from Colorado College and Zandra had returned from Alabama.

Ever since I had come back to Chicago after being fired by Pittsburgh, it became a tradition to celebrate Christmas at our home. We always have a Christmas Eve dinner at our place; Diana enjoys the planning and the cooking. When I was growing up, we always had Christmas at my parents' house, but they are getting a little older and it's just easier to do it at our house. We had about 17 in all, including Eddie's fiancée, Erika, as well as my brother Randy and his family.

Sadly, Lauren Graver, the young girl who participated with me in the ceremonial puck drop a month earlier at the United Center, passed away around Christmas time. In the obituary posted by the funeral home, Lauren was described as an inspiration to the community of Mount Prospect and beyond with the strength, bravery, and grace she displayed during her illness and that she brought out the best in people. To celebrate her life, it was suggested people wear what they felt best in, but noted Lauren would love it if her supporters wore the attire of her beloved Chicago Blackhawks. There were dozens of messages posted, some of them from people outside of Illinois who Lauren had emotionally touched.

A few weeks later I found a letter in my mailbox that must have been there awhile. It was from Lauren. It was really emotional to open that letter and read the note. Sometimes, life is truly unfair.

* * *

Early in the New Year, Pierre McGuire, one of my hockey broadcast partners on NBCSN, revealed publicly he had been diagnosed with prostate cancer back in the fall.

I called Pierre as soon as I heard and wished him well. When I got sick, Pierre texted me. It was like, what is happening with all of us getting cancer? Mike Milbury had a battle with kidney cancer, too, although he is 100 percent clean now. Enough already. Doc has often done public service announcements to talk about what he had gone through when diagnosed with Stage 1 prostate cancer in 1990 and to advocate for checkups.

Leading up to the Hawks' January 14 home game against Detroit, which would be televised on NBC and which I would be working, I was interviewed on the NHL Network by Jackie Redmond, E.J. Hradek, and Kevin Weekes. We talked about my health and hockey. I had just finished my ninth treatment and jokingly said it was not like I was counting but it was 40 days and six hours until I got unhooked. As I had in other interviews, I said I appreciated all the support from hockey fans, all the NHL teams, and everyone throughout the National Hockey League. The Philadelphia Flyers were incredible, in particular GM Ron Hextall. Team president Paul Holmgren, whom I have known for a long time, checked in and supported me. That meant a lot and it felt good to talk about hockey and provide insight into the struggling Hawks, which I noted was foreign territory for the team.

Around this time, I was in the shower and felt something the size of half a grapefruit above my belly button. Immediately I thought it was another tumor. I went to lie down and thankfully it went down, so I knew it wasn't a tumor. Then I began to think it was a hernia because I had had a sports hernia during my career around my crotch. It popped up and I pushed it in and it stayed in, but this one was higher, and when I stood up and pushed it in, it came back out.

I didn't want to self-diagnose, so I visited Dr. Terry and he confirmed it was a hernia. I looked pregnant. The hernia was another side effect and completely normal because the chemo eats away at the stitches on the inside and a hole develops, and that's dangerous because that's where your intestines are. When you develop a hole the size of a golf ball it becomes dangerous. But the doctors wouldn't let me have that fixed until I had a scan in March to see if I was cancer-free.

At the end of January, I participated from home in the inaugural Pegasus World Cup Betting Championship. The Pegasus is a thoroughbred race at Gulfstream Park in Florida that was conceived by track owner Frank Stronach and his daughter, Belinda, who collectively had the idea to make this the richest horse race in the world with a purse of $16 million, surpassing the $10 million Dubai World Cup. To be part of the betting challenge, participants had to pay a $12,000 entry fee for a chance to win a good chunk of the estimated $500,000 purse, which had a guaranteed pool of $300,000. The players with the highest amount of money accrued over the two-day tournament won. The results were posted online at Xpressbet.com.

In the media release announcing my participation, I talked about how the Pegasus is a unique, high-stakes tournament that brings together top horseplayers from around the world and how honored and excited I was to participate. I said that even though the field was loaded with exceptional handicappers, I would be shooting for the moon and had my sights set on finishing at the top of the leaderboard.

My strategy for tournament play was to commit to my convictions, manage my bankroll, and not be afraid to pick horses, regardless of their odds, if I thought they could win. That was the mistake I made in the 2016 Breeders' Cup Betting Challenge and it cost me. I wasn't going to repeat that mistake if I was in a position to win.

The rules for the two-day tournament on Gulfstream Park races stipulated players must bet a minimum total of $4,000 on Friday and must play at least five races. The following day, players had to bet a minimum of five races with a $1,000 minimum, and you had to bet a minimum of $3,000 on the Pegasus race.

I was sitting about 100th going into the final race of the 169 players who entered with $3,500. To me, the finish was ice cold. All I saw was Gun Runner, the 2017 Horse of the Year, winning and West Coast finishing second. I thought about picking a $3,000 exacta with my final bet, but that would have netted me about $25,000. The leaders had more than twice that amount. How do I turn an 8-1 shot into 50-1 or 60-1?

I zeroed in on Gunnevera and bet a $1,160 trifecta with Gun Runner, West Coast, and Gunnevera. I played some other combinations, including exactas with Gun Runner and West Coast, and some other trifectas with Gunnevera second just in case West Coast ran third.

Gun Runner, the heavy favorite, won easily, followed by West Coast. Gunnevera snuck in on the rail to finish third. I saw the trifecta paid $55.50 and began doing the math. I had at least $57,000 coming back. The leaders had about that amount going into the race and I didn't know how they played the race. I kept refreshing the page and called Hawks coach Joel Quenneville, who is a horse owner and horseplayer. He said he'd never heard of anybody betting a $1,100 trifecta.

I kept waiting and waiting and then, bam, it showed Eddie Olczyk on top with $65,858.20. Second-place finisher Tom Maloof had $62,294.

I got on the blower and called all my buddies: Dom, Joe the Judge, Coop, Joel, Jim Miller, Laffit Pincay III, and Double D (Darren Dunn of Assiniboia Downs in Winnipeg).

The first-place prize was $137,500, plus the money I won and an automatic invite to the 2018 Breeders' Cup Betting Challenge and the 2019 National Handicapping Competition.

I had talked to Darren Dunn earlier in the day about some of my strategies. His attitude is you don't win half a million dollars in a Pick 6 and more than $100,000 in a tournament if you're just throwing darts.

What I didn't know was that Gary Leeman, my linemate in Toronto, had been entered in the tournament with a friend and he couldn't believe I made a $1,100 straight trifecta bet. But I was in it to win it and didn't waver from my strategy.

I'd had a lot of medicine over the course of the last five months, but winning this tournament was the best medicine.

LAFFIT PINCAY III
NBC broadcaster

Part of why he was able to make such a strong comeback is he has such a strong, positive presence about him. In the end when he was able to walk away from this, that part really didn't surprise me, as scary and terrifying as it was when he was first diagnosed. Winning the Pegasus, I just knew how special that would be, that it was going to be the best medicine, in particular the way he did it from so far back, against the odds, and what he was dealing with from a health standpoint. I thought there was a parallel there; here's a guy who is going to come out swinging, fighting, and wind up on top.

Did I win because I'm a good handicapper or was it divine intervention because it made for a really good story? You need a little luck when handicapping, but I had learned from the 2017 Breeders' Cup Betting Challenge, in which I was in a really good spot, about 26th or 27th. All I saw was Arrogate and California Chrome and the rest of the field. I had more than enough money to do the bet, but I chickened out and bet a $4,000 exacta on Arrogate and California Chrome and bet $4,000 to win on Arrogate and a $300 trifecta and it came back $77. I would have won the tournament if I had followed my instincts. My attitude is, when playing in a tournament you can't be afraid to put your plums on the table. I wanted to make money in the Pegasus, but I really wanted to win the tournament.

I found out a few weeks later the victory meant I was eligible for a $1 million bonus if I won either the Breeders' Cup Betting Challenge or National Horseplayers Championship. So, this was like holding a lottery ticket.

I started to do more interviews to talk about my health, feeling it could help others going through their own cancer battles. In an interview I did with Matt Spiegel and Danny Parkins on *The Spiegel and Parkins Show* on 670 WSCR-AM, I talked about how my openness with my battle led to the early cancer detection and treatment for a radio listener's father.

"That is truly my inspiration and my goal," I said. "I know that I'm reaching out to people I don't know. The only reason I want to share my story is to help people. I'm trying to inspire one person to stay away from it or beat it themselves and hopefully it can be a domino effect down the road."

I said that I had 27 days to go until I was unhooked, hopefully for the last time, and put it in my rearview mirror.

"It's been a battle," I said. "It's hard to believe I'm down to the last four weeks. The last couple of months have been a grind. I'm just looking forward to getting back to what I love to do and that's doing hockey games and doing some horse racing and get back to some sort of normalcy and hopefully put this cancer behind me. Look, I'm still scared to death, that's for sure."

I talked about how I found out I'm tougher than I ever knew during the battle and I wanted cancer patients to know they are tough and strong, not weak, and that they will endure and conquer.

* * *

On February 21, at precisely 9:02 AM, I was unhooked from my final chemo treatment.

What a relief! It was incredible to be finally done—epic. I was done after six months. I had a bunch of family and friends call and congratulate me and I received so many texts from the hockey and horse racing worlds with exclamation points. Diana brought me a bouquet of helium balloons shaped like horses and dogs with the words You Did It. She almost flew away because of all the balloons.

After that last round of chemo, I got rid of anything that reminded me of what I had gone through during those treatments—clothes, pillows, blankets. Anything that reeked of chemo, I disposed of. That felt really good. The week before I went to the mall and went on a shopping spree. I was about to embark on the rest of my life and the rest of my career.

It was around this time that Illinois congressman Mike Quigley spoke on the House floor and addressed my situation. He had a Blackhawks jersey with my name and number brought in for display and talked about my battle and what I had been doing to raise awareness about the need for earlier screenings and continued research to find a cure. He described me as a native son of Chicago who has exemplified the heart, grit, and the character of the city we both call home.

"Like many others who have faced cancer, he was concerned that he was letting people down and he began to question his mortality, but as he went through treatment and reflected on this ordeal Eddie started to recognize that it was okay to be scared," Congressman Quigley said. "He knows it's important to emphasize that there's nothing wrong with people getting colonoscopies at an earlier age. He knows that if he can help just one individual get a checkup sooner, he will feel like his battle with cancer was worth it. To Eddie and to all fighting cancer, stay strong and know we're with you."

I was very grateful for him doing that. What an honor.

On March 8 I had the scan and the next day while traveling with the team to Boston, I asked Dr. Michael Terry, the Blackhawks team physician, if he had any update. He had been part of my illness from the start; I call him the captain of my doctors.

He had access to the scan on his iPhone. He looked at me and said, "Edzo, from what I can see, it looks really clean."

I gave him a huge hug because I'd just dodged a huge bullet. After getting emotional, I took a couple of deep breaths. I wanted to yell something like what most hockey players do after they score a goal, but I was just overcome thinking about so much—my family, my kids, my friends. I just couldn't wait to tell Diana that it looked good, but we still had to wait to hear from Dr. Mulcahy.

DR. MICHAEL TERRY
Blackhawks head team physician

It was one of those things where I didn't want to get in the way of the doctors managing him, but I also didn't want Eddie sitting there worried about it. Eddie was sitting across the aisle and one row back and he came over and asked me if I knew anything. When I told him everything looked negative, Eddie gave me a hug for about two minutes. That's the best news you can give somebody in that situation. Everybody loves Eddie Olczyk and everybody wants the best for him and certainly I did, too. I'm not going to tell you I was just as happy as he was, but I was close behind.

It was a relief and a half that it was all gone. Thank God. I was so thankful for the physicians and the team that I had and the support I had. It's always going to be with me, but I felt okay. We had come a long way since that first meeting with Dr. Mulcahy. Yes, it was absolute hell for six months. Going through the chemo was the most difficult part because there was a chance, God forbid, I'd have to continue with more treatment.

I endured a lot and tackled it straight on and felt like I had conquered it. Now I had to recover and rid myself of all this medicine and tell my story to encourage people to go in for checkups and get colonoscopies. This is why we tried to be so open and outgoing without being overbearing. If you don't feel good or you get to the age of 45, you've got to get checked, whether you have a history of cancer in your family or not.

I called Diana after we deplaned and told her the news and we subsequently gave the heads-up to the kids.

Four days later, at 5:07 PM, Dr. Mulcahy called and told me I was cancer-free. Diana was there with me and we didn't do anything special other than maybe hug a little tighter when I got back home. It was like, "We did it. Let's get as far away from this as we can."

On March 22, just before the start of the second period of a game at the United Center between the Hawks and the Vancouver Canucks, I went back on the air with Pat Foley to update people on my condition. He told the audience that because of what I had gone through, he had gotten a colonoscopy, as had Troy Murray and a bunch of Pat's friends. He said my ability to go public with what I had gone through was tremendously inspirational and also heroic, because anybody who has gone through chemotherapy knows how devastating a situation that can be.

Happily, I told everyone I was cancer-free. I reiterated as I had throughout my battle that it was a team effort, including the doctors, the entire Hawks organization, the National Hockey League, the people I worked with on TV, my family, my wife, my children, and my friends. If it wasn't for my family, there was no way I could have gone through this. We all beat this. And I said I had done enough crying to last me a lifetime.

Pat was so pumped. "You beat cancer, baby!" he exclaimed.

JOHN McDONOUGH
Blackhawks president and CEO

I was working out in the morning and he called me on my cell phone. During his treatment, I probably talked to him a couple of times a week. We kind of celebrated together. The call gave me an incredible bounce for the rest of that day, and quite frankly, the rest of the season. The next time I saw him it was very emotional and we hugged. We think he's an important part of our franchise. He's an ambassador. He's a liaison. He's somebody who kind of symbolizes our logo.

Now that I was publicly revealing I was cancer-free, I wanted to reinforce to people who were battling cancer or knew someone going through it that they are not weak individuals. My message for them was to stay strong, believe they are tough, and believe they will beat it. I ended the interview by saying if I could inspire one person to stay away from this by going for a colonoscopy, then I guess it was well worth it. It tests your will to live.

SAM FLOOD
NBC executive producer

I was in an executive meeting with all the leadership of NBC Universal. I got a call from Eddie during the meeting, which I didn't answer, and then a text that said, "Call me." I was thinking, holy crap, this is bad news. I walked out of the meeting—something you don't want to do with the big bosses—and called him. He said, "I'm cancer-free and I'm on a New York City street crying my eyes out." It's a moment I will never forget.

I did a bunch of interviews afterward, just as I had done since I went public with my cancer battle, so it was kind of like going full circle. It wasn't easy but it's a lot less stressful when you're telling them the happy ending of the story. Sharing that news was such a relief.

I subsequently underwent the hernia surgery in which they put an 8"x10" piece of mesh in my stomach to seal it up and fix it. In a way, it also felt like the final touch on my long journey.

CHAPTER 19

GETTING BACK ON THE BROADCASTING HORSE

I HAD ALREADY STARTED WORKING a regular broadcast schedule by the time of my hernia surgery and now the Stanley Cup playoffs were about to begin. The Kentucky Derby was about a month away. I would be working four to five days a week, but it was great to be back in the routine.

When I retired from playing, I missed my teammates. When I was going through my cancer battle, I missed the people I worked with and for. It's all about the people. When I returned it confirmed how much I love the people with whom I work. The skill of communicating and relationships is falling by the wayside because of social media and technology and I missed that camaraderie, whether it was an acquaintance or an old teammate or a coach or a writer or a trainer. That's what really got to me in a good way when I got back to working full time.

One of the last goals I set for myself was to be well enough to work the entire Triple Crown series and the Stanley Cup Final. The Derby is the first Saturday in May and I arrived in Kentucky four days before the race. The last race I had worked for NBC before I was diagnosed with cancer was the Belmont Invitational in New York the previous July. That was kind of like an appetizer before I really got back into the regular horse racing routine.

There are a lot more people working the Triple Crown and the outreach was overwhelming. It was just great to be back, just like when I was getting back into hockey broadcasting again. Seeing a lot of horsemen and having them tell me they were happy I was back and healthy meant the world to me. It felt good, especially after having gone through the hell of cancer and chemotherapy.

On our Friday broadcast for the Kentucky Oaks, which is the Derby for three-year-old fillies, it was tough sledding with my picks. I learned that humility is a skill as well and I think I've been able to display that my whole life, especially when on TV. But Oaks day was fair warning. If it was a one-horse race I'd have still lost. We had some fun with that on the broadcast with fellow announcer Jerry Bailey jokingly busting my balls. But that's betting; sometimes it goes like that.

The Derby was a wild experience because it was raining like crazy on the day of the race, the most rainfall in the race's history, which began in 1875. There were a couple of inches of rain on the track. Aside from my job handicapping the race, I also did the walkover with the horses and the horsemen on the track en route to the paddock. I interviewed trainer Todd Pletcher, who had Audible, Noble Indy, Vino Rosso, and Magnum Moon in the field of 20, the maximum number of starters. There was mud everywhere, and when you're doing that interview it's pretty intense. There are hundreds of people around, 1,200-pound animals, and trainers who are focused on a lot of things. You're walking and talking and you don't want to teakettle it, either. That's the biggest fear. Tripping would make for great TV—it would be on the Internet forever—so it's really intense.

The hot horse going into the race was trainer Bob Baffert's Justify, who had not started as a two-year-old but had won all three races as a three-year-old. I had been in California for the broadcast of the Santa Anita Derby, a major Derby prep. The last time a horse won the Derby

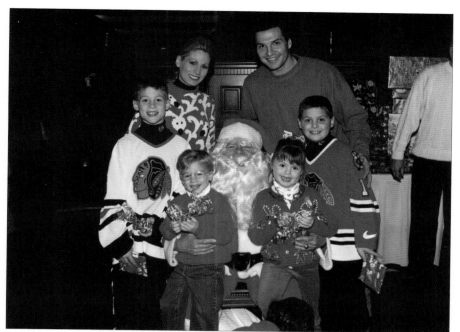

Diana and I with Santa and the kids. From left: Eddie, Nick, Zandra, and Tommy.

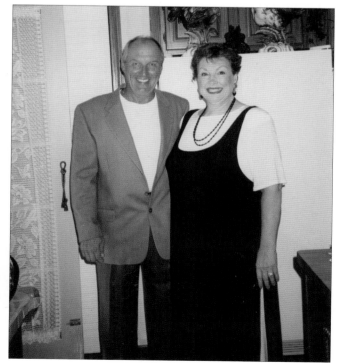

My parents, Ed and Diana.

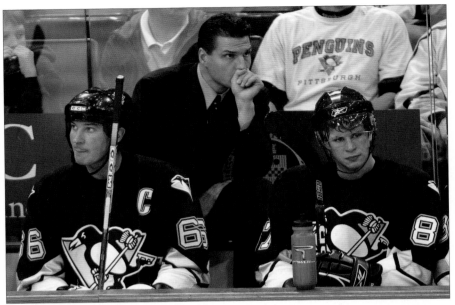

It was a privilege to coach Mario Lemieux and Sidney Crosby in Pittsburgh. I'm disappointed I wasn't able to see it through but not in a million years do I regret taking the job. (Getty Images)

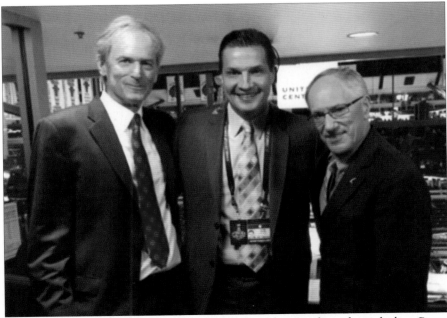

I've had the opportunity to work with some broadcasting legends, including Pat Foley (left) and Doc Emrick (right). We have each other's back in and out of the booth.

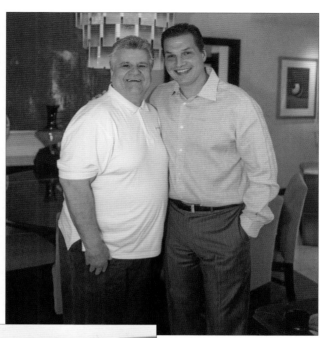

Me and my buddy, Dominic Porro.

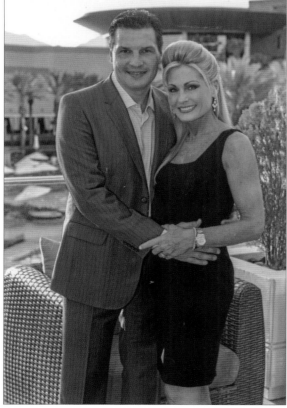

Me and Diana. She is the strongest person I've ever known.

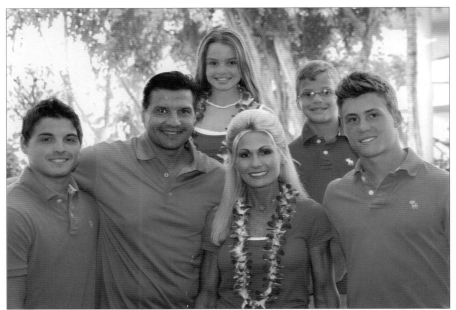

On vacation in Hawaii when the kids were a little younger. From left: Tommy, Zandra, Nick, and Eddie.

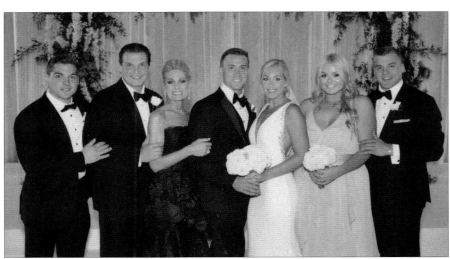

Eddie and Erika's wedding day was one of those dates I had circled on my calendar. From left: Tommy, me, Diana, Eddie, Erika, Zandra, and Nick.

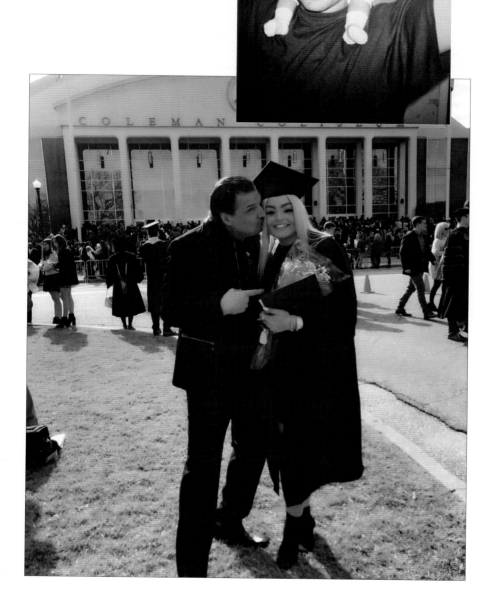

Where has the time gone? With Zandra as a baby (top) and at her graduation from the University of Alabama (bottom).

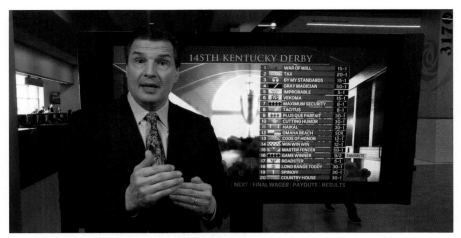

I'll be forever grateful to NBC's Sam Flood for making me a part of NBC's coverage of horse racing. At the 145th Kentucky Derby (top) and at the 2019 Royal Ascot in the United Kingdom (below). (NBC)

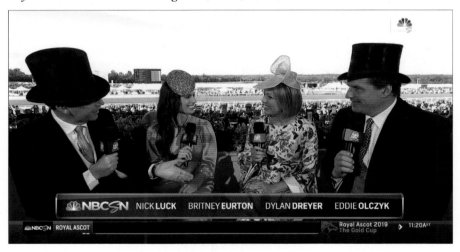

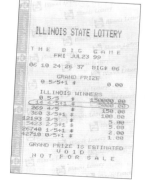

Talk about beating the odds! Dom and I were one number away from winning $80 million in the Illinois lottery.

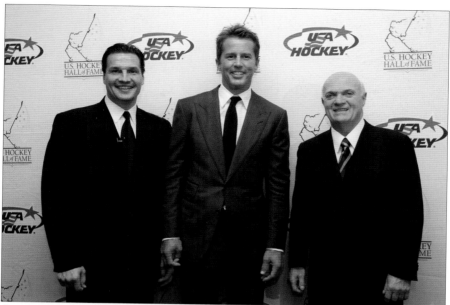

It was truly humbling to be inducted into the U.S. Hockey Hall of Fame alongside Mike Modano and Lou Lamoriello. (AP Images)

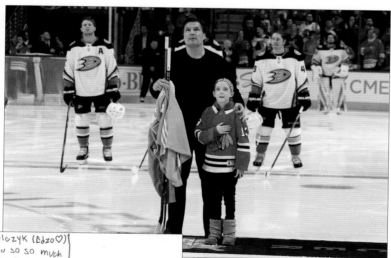

Dear Mr. Oloczyk (Edzo♡),
Thank you so so much for an unforgettible night. I felt so honored to drop the puck with you. And just as I thought the night couldn't get any better, you gave me your jersey. I love the jersey so much! You are a true hero and we pray for you every day. Thanks for a night I won't forget.

Love, your friend forever, Lauren Graver

With Lauren Graver at the United Center during Hockey Fights Cancer night in 2018. A few weeks after she passed, I found a letter she'd written me in my mailbox (inset). Sometimes, life is truly unfair. (Getty Images)

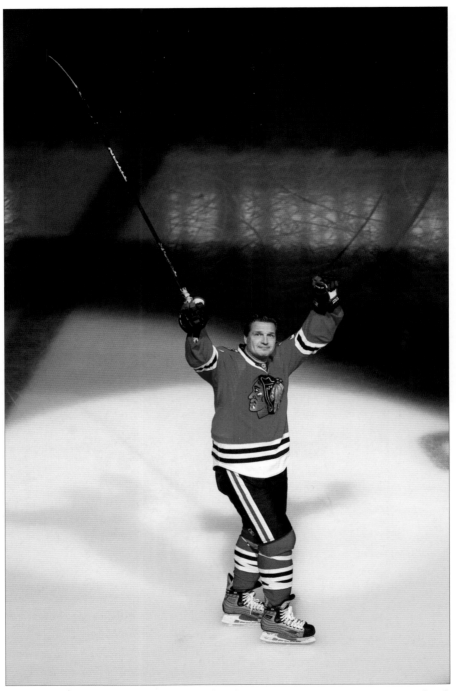

One More Shift, courtesy of the Blackhawks in 2018. It was a great way to thank the team, the fans, and the game of hockey for everything they've given me.
(AP Images)

that hadn't run in a race as a two-year-old happened back in 1882. I liked Good Magic, trained by Chad Brown, who had won the champion two-year-old honors. Good Magic had raced twice going into the Derby, finishing third by 2 lengths in his season debut and winning his next by 1½ lengths. My third choice was Audible, who had won four of five career races. I liked Good Magic because the price was right at 9-1 and he was a little more seasoned than Justify, would get a good trip, and liked the off track. A sloppy track is the great equalizer. Some horses thrive on an off track particularly if they are frontrunners and aren't getting mud thrown back in their faces, and some just can't handle it. With a full field of relatively young, inexperienced horses anything can happen. I wasn't sure if Good Magic could last the distance of a mile and a quarter, but thought I'd go with him because the odds were good and hope he could beat the favorite.

I said on the air I was going to box Good Magic, Justify, and Audible in various trifecta combinations. You can bet a $1 tri box, which costs $6, or a $2 tri box for $12. I was also boxing Good Magic and Justify for the exacta, which costs $4. Justify went postward as the race favorite at just under 3–1, while Audible was 7-1.

Justify ran close to the pacesetter Promises Fulfilled, a 48-1 long shot, and seized the lead after one mile by 1½ lengths over Good Magic. Justify opened up his lead in the stretch and Good Magic was laboring. Meanwhile, Audible started to make a huge move from far back to third. I knew Good Magic wasn't going to catch Justify, who proved to be a beast, but at that point I thought I had a chance to hit the trifecta. Justify won comfortably by 2½ lengths over Good Magic, who finished second by a head over Audible.

It was raining pretty hard in the paddock and I had to keep an eye on Todd because I had to interview him if one of his horses won, but at the finish I was celebrating like I had just scored a goal. All of us on the broadcast give out our picks and I'm considered the expert. To stand up there in front of millions of people watching the race worldwide and pick the top three felt great. Everybody who bets on horse races has an opinion and when you are on TV, especially in that setting, you are talking to a lot of people who don't regularly watch horse racing or only watch the Kentucky Derby or the Triple Crown races. When I pick the winner or give out the trifecta, it builds credibility. There's no doubt about that. No one is going to remember my pick for some big races that are not part of the Triple Crown except the diehard racing fans, but to accomplish that on the biggest stage of the year makes everything else gravy. It felt so good, especially not knowing a few months back if I was even going to be healthy enough to be at the Derby. It probably meant a little bit more to pick the trifecta than any other winners that I've picked.

I cashed about $28,000 after investing $1,800. You've got people on Wall Street trying to make 3 or 4 percent of their money on a day. I know it's different betting horses, but there still is that gambling, risk-taking part of it. If Good Magic could have beaten Justify—and we all know what ifs are worth—I could have won $100,000. That would have been a humongous score because the majority of my tickets had Good Magic on top, but that's horse racing. Giving out the trifecta on national TV meant even more than cashing my ticket.

Okay, not really. I wanted to stuff my pockets and add to my Xpressbet account. It was like the bases were loaded with two out and we were down by two and I drove in all three runs. It's great to go to the window and go to my Xpressbet account and see it ring up, but like I said I did my job and hopefully people watched and cashed. I've had people thank me because they played my numbers and that's great because it's why I'm there.

I returned back to my broadcasting duties and was working on Mother's Day and took that occasion to thank my mother for all she had done to help me pursue my hockey dreams. I had promised my mom and Diana during my cancer battle that I would be with them for Mother's Day. So even though I wasn't physically there with them that day, I was there in spirit. I wanted the hockey world to know that both of them helped me through a really tough time and that I loved them. I got emotional and my NBC studio broadcast partner Keith Jones said, "I'm glad you spent it with me and don't make me cry." That made me laugh. Jonesy is the best, a great colleague and a great friend. If I am ever in a pinch, I know Jonesy would have my back—and he loves the ponies, too.

I was back the following week in Baltimore for the Preakness Stakes, the second leg of the Triple Crown. Once again it was raining and I picked Justify to win and Good Magic to finish second. I thought nobody could run with Justify because he was proven on an off track. This time I didn't have to walk over the muddy track with the horsemen and the horses.

Justify and Good Magic ran eyeball to eyeball for most of the opening three quarters of the mile-and-three-sixteenths race. As this was happening, I was thinking, there's no way Good Magic could beat Justify, who was the 2-5 betting favorite. Justify won by a half-length over 15-1 long shot Bravazo, followed a neck back by 26-1 long shot Tenfold. Good Magic, who was the second choice in the wagering at just under 4-1 odds, finished a close fourth. I did not like the ride Good Magic got and I thought it cost him a better placing. Hall of Fame jockey Jerry Bailey disagreed with me. Oh, well.

I played trifectas and exactas with Good Magic second and third. It's tough to make any money on a horse that has such low odds. Overall, I had a good weekend with my picks.

Three weeks later in New York for the Belmont Stakes, there was tremendous excitement because of the possibility of a Triple Crown sweep. This was my fourth year working the Triple Crown for NBC and I had a chance to witness my second Triple Crown sweep. American Pharoah did it in 2015, and here I was with a chance to witness history again. It was never going to be like American Pharoah because it was the unknown of whether he could do it. With Justify, I was convinced he was going to do it, so my excitement was tempered a bit this time.

The race attracted 10 starters because despite the fact Justify was the overwhelming choice to win, the purse was still $1.5 million. While it would be great for horse racing to have another Triple Crown winner, horsemen weren't going to hand him the win. It was a still a horse race and history has proven time and time again that anything can happen.

This time it was a sunny day and the track was fast and dry. Justify was the 4-5 favorite to win the race. Tenfold and Bravazo were the only other horses that had run in the Preakness. One of the horses was Gronkowski, named after New England Patriots tight end Rob Gronkowski, who was one of the colt's owners.

Jockey Mike Smith took Justify immediately to the front and was never seriously challenged and won by 1¾ lengths. It was absolutely incredible to see that history again three years after American Pharoah. Gronkowski, who was a long shot at almost 25-1 odds, ran second, followed by Hofburg, a 6-1 shot, which had run in the Derby. Neither Tenfold nor Bravazo were a factor.

I couldn't lose on Friday with my picks and on Saturday I didn't do anything of significance. Tough day on Black Rock on Saturday. It goes like that. When I have a bad day handicapping, I'm not happy about it, especially when I'm doing it for TV. But as I said, humility is a good quality to have, as is being able to make fun of yourself.

At the NBC compound after the race, I saw Sam Flood, who was talking to his wife, Jane. Everyone was so pumped about the show and seeing history and I pulled him off to the side and said, "I've been with you guys for four years of NBC's Triple Crown coverage and we've had two Triple Crowns." I was of course taking some credit.

Without hesitation, as only Sam could do, he said, "Well, what happened with the other two?"

* * *

Once the Triple Crown was over, it was back to the Stanley Cup playoffs, which had some surprises.

I thought before it started the Nashville Predators and Tampa Bay Lightning would battle it out for the Cup, but neither made it to the

Final. Nashville lost to the Winnipeg Jets in the Western Conference semifinals, while Tampa Bay lost to the Washington Capitals in the Eastern Conference Final. I had a soft spot for the city of Winnipeg and the franchise because of my five years playing for the Jets and the painful memory of seeing the team forced to leave because of financial reasons. I knew the fan base and the pulse of the city and what it would mean for the Jets to win the Cup.

On October 22, 2016, I played for the Jets against the Edmonton Oilers as part of the Heritage Classic alumni game, played outdoors at Investors Group Field in Winnipeg. It was an honor and a privilege to be part of the game, and wearing the Jets jersey with my name on the back brought back so many memories of my time in the Peg.

I had been part of 10 or so NHL outdoor games, but this was different because it was played in the fall and I was part of an alumni game that preceded a regular season game. The Oilers lineup included several players who were teammates of mine on the New York Rangers' 1994 Stanley Cup team. During the '80s, the Jets routinely faced the Oilers, who were captained by Wayne Gretzky, and couldn't get by them in the playoffs. The alumni game was broadcast on the CBC and it was a great experience. We won the game 6–5 on a penalty shot by Teemu Selanne with only a few seconds left in the third period.

There was a one in four chance of the Jets winning the Cup in these playoffs, but like any team at that point they would need a combination of luck and healthy bodies. The Jets lost to the expansion Vegas Golden Knights in five games in the Western Conference Final. I still believe the Jets will win the Cup at some point.

Few people would have expected the Golden Knights to make the playoffs, let alone the Final. They became the feel-good story of the season and in all of sports, trying to make history and become the first expansion team to win the Cup.

Was it cool to see Vegas in the Final? Everybody who knows me knows that is the wrong question to ask. It's like, hey, I'm going to Vegas to work a hockey game. And by the way, the games all start at 5:00 PM local time and I'll be done by 8:00 and have plenty of time to do what I want to do.

The Caps started out the playoffs losing their opening two games in overtime at home to the Columbus Blue Jackets and desperately needed to win the third game, which they did in double overtime. They also won the fifth game in overtime. The main reason they won is because they checked better than anyone else. That's not sexy and I don't think people thought of the Capitals as a checking team, so that's what was so remarkable about what they did. They overcame some adversity and the right team won. They were down against Columbus, they beat the Pittsburgh Penguins—who had won the last two Cups—and they rallied back to win the final two games against Tampa after winning the first two games and losing the next three. They finished it off beating Vegas after losing the opening game of the series. Every time you turned around, everyone was trying to put a cement block in front of the Caps, but they always overcame it.

It was a redemption of sorts for Capitals captain Alexander Ovechkin, who had been criticized in the media as a great player who had not done well in the Stanley Cup playoffs and Olympics. He silenced his critics with a solid performance in the Final. It's great when superstar players win the Cup because of the attention it gets for our game. You need the studs and a little luck, but when the door is open you've got to take advantage of it.

As for Vegas, in my opinion they were not only the sports team of the year but the sports team of the decade, too. The team wasn't even around 10 months before that and it was absolutely great to see what they accomplished. Look at all the sports that had expansion teams come in and they were all doormats for the most part. To see a team do what they did and go as far as they did in a city like Vegas, it was just absolutely incredible. It was not normal. I don't care what sport it is. Seeing history being made with Justify and seeing what Vegas was on the verge of doing and everything else, it was just an incredible story.

* * *

The Chicago Cubs invited me to throw out the first pitch and sing "Take Me Out to the Ball Game" at a home game in July. It wasn't the first time I had thrown out the first pitch—I had done it once before—but this meant so much more.

I was more nervous about throwing out the first pitch than singing. The worse you are singing that song, the better it is, I guess. It was my fifth time singing at a Cubs game. My kids were busting my chops that I better throw it all the way to the plate and not bounce it. Diana and all of the kids were there except Eddie, who was away coaching. Cubs pitcher Mike Montgomery was behind the plate to catch the ball. I had fans at the game tell me I had to throw from the mound and not from a few feet in front of it. So, there I was on the mound with thousands of people watching in the stadium and many more watching on TV and all I could think was, don't bounce it, don't bounce it, don't bounce it.

We have the two Labs at home and I throw the tennis ball for them hundreds of times a week. My arm was well-oiled. Throwing a baseball and a tennis ball aren't exactly the same thing, but it's not like I haven't thrown a ball in 15 or 20 years. I wound up and threw a fastball that bent late right across the heart of the plate. Mike said I had a little cut to the pitch and I told him it was with the seams. It was a lot of fun.

I love baseball. I always have. It didn't matter where I laced my skates as a hockey player. I'd go to baseball games wherever I was. I went to a lot of Blue Jays games in Toronto when I was with the Leafs, and in New York when I played for the Rangers and in Los Angeles when I played for the Kings, and obviously I've been a Cubs fan my whole life. To get that chance again was great. Mike and I signed the ball and I gave it to a young fan in the crowd. It was just a great experience.

Independent of the pitch, it was great to be there and do it after what I had been through. The fans were great, really loud, in welcoming me. It was hard not to think about what Pat did back in September. I tried to continue to be an inspiration to people with cancer and help them find the will and the want to battle every day. Maybe I inspired somebody being there.

Before I sang, I spent some time with Len Kasper and J.D.—Jim Deshaies—the Cubs TV broadcasters, and Pat Hughes and Ron Coomer on the radio side. They are just great guys. The Cubs treated us great.

I was interviewed a few days later by Jamie Hersch and E.J. Hradek on the NHL Network and was asked about the experience, in particular the singing. I jokingly said there's a show called *America's Got Talent* and I belonged on *America's Got No Talent*.

I emceed the Hawks' 11th annual Blackhawks Convention week and that again proved to be emotional. I introduced Pat, who was sitting in the crowd and joined me, and the crowd shouted, "Edd-ie, Edd-ie, Edd-ie." That meant a lot and it was a chance again to express my love and thank everyone who had helped me in my battle. It was so emotional and I cried, but I repeated I had done enough crying the last 11 months to last me a lifetime.

CHAPTER 20

A BLESSED UNION

EDDIE MARRIED ERIKA BOZIN on August 4, a year to the day after I was diagnosed with cancer. It was another one of those dates I had circled on my calendar. I planned to be there in sickness or in health, and fortunately I was well.

The wedding took place at the Four Seasons Hotel in downtown Chicago. The Royal Wedding between Prince Harry and Meghan Markle had nothing on this one. The Kardashians would probably learn a thing or two from it. It was beautiful, a great celebration, for sure. There was nothing that was missed, no oversights.

Diana and I were responsible for organizing the rehearsal dinner the night before at Chicago Cut Steakhouse, which was attended by 125 guests. Erika's parents, Chris and Kristie Bozin, organized the wedding. They get full credit for putting on an incredible evening.

The experience of seeing your first child marry brought back so many memories. Where has the time gone? Bringing him into this world in Toronto 29 years ago, watching him grow up and play baseball and hockey, moving around like we did, going to college at the University of Massachusetts–Amherst, playing a little minor pro in the Southern League and then coaching...and then all of a sudden, he's getting married? I got married when I was 21. You just sit there and realize, man, it's way too fast. I would give anything that I have or earned to go back 10 years with my kids. Obviously, I know that can't happen. I wouldn't treat them any differently or give them more. It's just the actual act of watching your kids grow up and really missing the innocence of a young person. As kids we want to grow up and become teenagers and then adults. You want to hurry, but you're going to do enough hurrying when you get old. That's life.

Diana and I tried to prioritize being around as much as we could as parents. Look, sometimes work prevents that. Sometimes sickness prevents that. Sometimes life prevents that and you've got to make the effort and that's what I always tried to do, whether it was taking the kids to school, even when I was playing, or being at one of their events. There were lots of times I couldn't be in places, but it's like any other family member that is providing for the family. There's give and take.

I really believe home is where you learn about life and discipline. If you ask any of my kids if they grew up in a relaxed environment or a strict environment, I'm sure they would all say it was very strict—too strict, I am sure. There was lots of respect and there were rules, but there was a lot of love and support. Having dinner as a family, those are the things that are important.

The one thing that I've always emphasized with Diana and the people who are very close and important to me is how I feel about them and how thankful and appreciative I am of them. I would never want to have left this earth and not have them know how much they mean to me. Life's too short, but I would be really devastated if someone I loved or cared about didn't know what they meant to me.

I told Eddie and Erika to let them know how much they mean to one another. Despite how crazy and busy life is, make sure you go out of your way to let each other know how important they are. You're going to have arguments, you're going to disagree, you're going to be angry, but don't go to bed angry. You can be disappointed, but when you put your head on the pillow at night just make sure you are communicating and you respect one another. That's something I learned from my parents and something I've tried to emulate.

I'm sure for Eddie it probably wasn't always easy being Eddie Olczyk. I named him Eddie out of respect for my dad. But on the night of his wedding, we were all proud he was Eddie Olczyk.

It's an emotional time as a parent. I remember when Eddie was a baby he had a pacifier that he could spin like you wouldn't believe. It was like a top in his mouth. I was worried he was going to fly away a couple of times because he was moving it so fast. I don't know how he did it. Where the hell did that time go?

It was a great celebration. We love Erika and her family is terrific. They live about a driver and a wedge away from our house. We've known each other for a long, long time. Eddie and Erika went their separate ways for a long time, but we always thought they were meant for each other and eventually they found each other again and the rest is history.

I'm sure for Diana it was special seeing her first child getting married, but it was hard for her after losing her mom a few years earlier. It's emotional on a lot of different levels. You love all your kids unconditionally, but to see your first child get married gets the blood pumping, for sure.

Tommy and Nicky were the co-best men, and Zandra was one of the bridesmaids. It was truly a family affair. Tommy and Nicky both spoke at the wedding. To see them walking down the aisle had me remembering pushing strollers, caring for them, putting on their skates, and taking them to school. Now here they were as adults, watching their brother get married and entering into a new family and bringing a new member into our family. It was quite the experience.

Diana and I went to Las Vegas to celebrate our 30th anniversary. We've been going there for about 15 years and stay at the Red Rock Casino Resort and Spa. It's located 150 yards away from the Golden Knights' practice facility in a suburb called Summerlin, which is about 12 miles outside the strip. We'll go into town for a show or dinner, but I'm a little too old for the strip. I like the racebook and the steakhouse—T-Bones

Chophouse—at the Red Rock Resort. Jason McCormick, the director of race and sports, is a Chicago guy and takes incredible care of us. We do our thing. It's just been a constant in our life to go there, hang out, and not live by any schedules.

It felt so good to be getting back to normal.

CHAPTER 21

ONE MORE SHIFT

IN THE MONTHS AFTER it was determined I was free of cancer, there were some things that happened that made me appreciate how lucky I am to be healthy.

In October 2018, I received the National Hockey League Alumni Association Ace Bailey Award of Courage. The award, named for the Los Angeles Kings scout who died in the 9/11 terrorist attacks, is given annually to a recipient who has shown exceptional courage and exemplary determination in life.

I talk to Glenn Healy, the executive director of the alumni association, quite often and when he called to tell me about the award I thought he was busting my balls. That's just the relationship we have. Heals has done an amazing job since being appointed in June 2017. We played together in New York when we won the Cup in 1994 and for a few weeks in the minors with the Chicago Wolves in 1998. He's been more than a great teammate over the years; he's been a great human being and somebody I respect a whole lot. He's made a great impact on me. When he told me about the gala and that I was to be the recipient of the award, I was taken aback and humbled. I couldn't have been prouder to be chosen.

The event took place in Toronto and when I entered the building for the cocktail reception the first person I saw was Rick Vaive, who was traded to Chicago in the deal that brought me to Toronto in 1987. Then

I ran into Tie Domi, who had been traded to Winnipeg in the deal that brought me to New York in 1992. And then I saw Steve Thomas, who was involved with Vaive in the Chicago deal, and this string of coincidences continued with Kris King, who was part of the Domi deal. It was like everyone I saw was part of a trade in my career. I was beginning to think there was a hidden camera somewhere and this was an Eddie Olczyk *This Is Your Life* episode involving all my trades. I mentioned that in my acceptance speech.

The assembled crowd included NHL commissioner Gary Bettman—who checked up on me when I was sick—deputy commissioner Bill Daly, and NHL Players Association executive director Don Fehr. There were also teammates from my Stanley Cup year in New York, such as Adam Graves and Heals. Hawks broadcasters Troy Murray and Pat Foley came in for the event and that made it even more special.

Behind the speaker's podium were old photos of Bobby Hull when he played for the Blackhawks and Gordie Howe with Detroit. Since I began telling my story to audiences, I've tried to make an impact on the people I am addressing. In this case it was the alumni, many of whom were my age.

You could hear a pin drop and feel the power and emotion in the room when I was speaking. I could see some people were emotional. I was just trying to tell my story of where I had been and where I was trying to get to. I wanted the people there to know one day I woke up in a bad situation and the disease tested my will to live, but that I was not afraid to ask for help and found out I was much stronger than I ever knew.

GLENN HEALY
NHL Alumni Association executive director

When we picked Eddie for the 2018 Ace Bailey Courage Award, there wasn't a second choice. It was one guy, Eddie. In the speech he gave at our gala, there wasn't anybody not crying in the room, and there were some alpha personalities there, guys who had armor around them. I expected that type of speech because Eddie carried himself with such grace and poise and dignity in his career, that when faced with this I knew he was going to do it with those same qualities.

I have shared my personal journey many times with a vast number of audiences, but some people may not have heard it. Each opportunity I get to speak can be educational, informative, and, more than anything, personal. I'm trying to reach as many people as possible through the platforms and opportunities that I have since I went public with my story.

In November 2018 the Blackhawks honored me with One More Shift, something they had done for alumni to allow fans to recognize them one final time by skating in full uniform on the ice at a home game before the playing of the national anthem. The list of players who have been honored started with Denis Savard and includes Bryan Bickell, Al Secord, Eric Daze, Troy Murray, Stan Mikita, Steve Larmer, Jeremy Roenick, and Ed Belfour.

When I had seen former players do it, it was pretty remarkable. What a way to connect the current fan base with the past. A lot of fans probably have no idea who I am, let alone that I played as long as I did. I always wondered if I'd ever be a guy who gets One More Shift.

The more I thought about this incredible opportunity, the more I realized this was finally going to give me some closure on my NHL career. Remember, when I retired in 2000, Mike Smith had no interest in allowing me to retire as a Blackhawk. I had that conversation with Hawks president/CEO John McDonough and I don't think John realized how special this was going to be for me. I always wished I'd had that chance. Now it was going to happen—just 18-plus years later.

The closure was my way of thanking the game, thanking the fans, and thanking the Blackhawks for five years of my playing career for Chicago and 16 years in the NHL.

My parents were there along with my brother Randy. Diana was in Paris with Zandra visiting Tommy, who was playing in France. Eddie was away coaching and Nicky was in school.

The ceremony began with images from my playing career displayed on the giant scoreboard, accompanied by the song "Blue Collar Man" by Styx. There were also images of myself projected on the ice before I was introduced as "Chicago's own Eddie Olczyk."

As I began the skate, the crowd cheered and members of both the Hawks and visiting Minnesota Wild clapped and tapped their sticks against the boards. I didn't see any of the images of myself on the ice because I was looking at the crowd with my stick raised. I was in a daze. I had already been told in a good-natured way by about 500 people not to fall, including team owner Rocky Wirtz and John McDonough.

I then skated over to the Hawks starters—Patrick Kane, Corey Crawford, Brandon Saad, Jonathan Toews, Duncan Keith, and Brent Seabrook—and said a few words to them. Kane and Seabrook asked if I had a shift or two in me. I said maybe a faceoff and a power-play shift, but other than that I got nothing. I then skated over to the team's bench to acknowledge the players and coaches. I especially wanted to see head athletic trainer Mike Gapski, whom I call Frank because he walks like Frankenstein, head equipment manager Troy Parchman, and massage therapist Pawel Prylinski. They were all there when I played my last game in the NHL against the St. Louis Blues in 2000. It kind of took me back 18 years. Seeing all those guys again was awesome.

I was in the ceremonial faceoff with Carter Holmes, an 11-year-old boy from Viroqua, Wisconsin, who was battling Hodgkin's lymphoma and was appearing in conjunction with the Make-A-Wish Foundation. Wild captain Mikko Koivu participated with me in the faceoff. His brother, Saku, had successfully battled non-Hodgkin's lymphoma while captain of the Montreal Canadiens in 2001. I must have taken 100 draws against Saku during my career and didn't win any of them, so when I saw Mikko coming over I told him I had to win this faceoff because his brother owned me in my playing days. I wasn't going to lose this last one. I don't think he understood what I saying to him, but I went old school as soon as Carter dropped the puck and slashed Mikko's stick and pulled the puck back and won the draw. I gave the puck to Carter and Mikko gave him his stick. After it was all over, I returned to the press box and resumed the broadcast.

Collectively it was way more than I thought it would be. I finally had closure.

JOHN McDONOUGH
Blackhawks president and CEO

We introduced the concept of One More Shift about three years ago. It's a very dignified and respectful way of saluting the careers of players who played an important part in our franchise. So when I told Eddie about it, I think it put an exclamation point on his career. I think it's something he was overwhelmed with. From a timing standpoint, it couldn't have been better. I think Eddie was extremely flattered. Going around the ice like that, it's very dramatic.

On the Blackhawks website, Bob Verdi, who had covered so many of my games as a columnist with the *Chicago Tribune*, wrote, "Forever it seems Eddie Olczyk has been referred to in several ways by friends and fans who are fonder of him than trying to spell his last name. Edzo. Eddie. Eddie O. But on Sunday, as if to close the book and post results of his fight against a relentless foe, you wanted to put a final score on the board. Eddie 1, Cancer 0."

What a line from Verdi. I've known him a long time, he's a brilliant writer, and it brought a few tears to my eyes. Whether he's writing about hockey or golf or just about any subject, he's got a way with words.

CHAPTER 22

A RANGERS REUNION

THE FOLLOWING FEBRUARY I attended the New York Rangers' 25th anniversary celebration of the 1994 Stanley Cup win. It took place over the course of a few days in New York and most everyone associated with the team was thinking, where in the hell did 25 years go?

It's never the same as when you are in the moment and going through the playoff run and then celebrating and the subsequent days and weeks after. But you never lose that bond and respect and appreciation for what we did. We've lost some people along the way, whether it was training staff or Alexander Karpovtsev, who died in 2011 in the Lokomotiv Yaroslavl plane crash that killed members of the team playing in the Kontinental Hockey League. He was an assistant coach of the team.

We had dinner at a restaurant called Lavo for families, friends, and guests on the first night of the festivities. It was a great chance to sit down with guys I hadn't seen in a while and find out what's going on. In true hockey form, you always get back to the hockey part of it and talk about stories that happened in the locker room or on the bus or on the bench. The next night the guys got together early in the day and then had a bunch of things to do at Madison Square Garden for season-ticket holders and media. We then had a ceremony before the start of the game, in which the Rangers were hosting the Carolina Hurricanes, and an after-party. It was a full two-plus days of activities before everyone left.

Mike Keenan was there. Every time I've seen him it's always cordial and respectful. I still have those raw feelings from when he was the coach of the team and decided I would be a role player no matter how hard I tried to convince him I could be a regular player. But you live and learn and you never forget. When I got cancer he never reached out, which is fine. Did I expect him to? I don't know. The difference between him and me is that when I found out he was diagnosed with prostate cancer in September 2018 and went public with it, I reached out to him. Right or wrong, I did.

Before the actual ceremony I was with Mike Hartman, Joey Kocur, Doug Lidster, and Jay Wells, and Mike came by. We were telling stories and yukking it up and he asked me if I was wearing alligator shoes—a reference to the comments he made to me 25 years ago. Everyone had a quick chuckle over it. Other than that, there was no drama.

The players were paraded out in numerical order, except for the captain and alternate captain, who went last. I was introduced by Sam Rosen and John Davidson, the TV voices for the Rangers in 1994. Both of them are great people who took a real interest in my battle with cancer. Sam still does play-by-play for the team today, and J.D. is back as team president. They made reference to the Players' Player Award I received at the end of the regular season for my contributions to the team. The fans were rhythmically shouting "Let's Go Rangers" and clapping their hands. It was pretty amazing. The Rangers organization did an amazing job with the weekend.

There hasn't been a time in all my years traveling to New York or the tri-state area, whether I was playing at the end of my career, broadcasting in the early 2000s, coaching in Pittsburgh, or broadcasting full time since 2006, that a Rangers fan hasn't approached me to say, "Thanks for '94" or "Heave-ho." That means a lot. We had a huge impact on the city bringing that Cup to New York to end a 54-year drought. My role was very small on that team, but when you are a part of a team and you accept your role to the best of your abilities, you are very much at peace.

For a brief second as I walking out on to the ice, I thought about where I was at this point a year ago and was just thankful to be alive. I was so lucky to have been a small part of a team that won it all and was there to enjoy the moment after my illness.

The reunion was everything I thought it would be. It brought back a lot of memories, a lot of stories, and was a genuinely great experience. The Rangers did an amazing job and it was nice to see familiar faces and talk about the past. I experienced a wide range of emotions. You're celebrating something that happened and who knows what is going to happen tomorrow, let alone 10 or 15 or 25 years from now. It was great to see guys and find out what's going on in their daily lives. Alex Kovalev came from China where he is working. Esa Tikkanen came from Finland. Kevin Lowe and Craig MacTavish came from Edmonton. There's a bunch of guys still living in the New York area. But no matter where we live, we'll all be bonded together forever.

CHAPTER 23

WITNESSING HISTORY (AGAIN)

GOING INTO THE 2019 KENTUCKY DERBY and anticipating a sloppy track, I liked Omaha Beach. He was the 4-1 morning-line favorite, but he was scratched three days before the race with a throat ailment that required surgery. I had Roadster in my Derby future book bet, meaning I bet him early and locked in my price, hoping for a bigger price than he would be at the Derby. I wagered $200 apiece at 24-1 and 16-1. I made these wagers based on a fast, sunny track.

One of the storylines going into the race was Maximum Security. His owners, Mary and Gary West, bred the colt and ran him for the first time in a $16,000 maiden claiming race. To put that in perspective, someone could have bought him for $16,000 before the race and owned what became a major contender for the Derby, although no one could have predicted that then. I'm pretty sure the Wests or trainer Jason Servis did not know what kind of a colt they had at that point. Running in a $16,000 maiden claiming race and going on to win the Florida Derby and having a Derby contender is the stuff you dream about as an owner. Just goes to show, whether it's a first-round draft pick in the NHL or the last pick, anything is possible. The Wests have pumped millions of dollars into the business, but they had never won the Derby.

When rain started to fall leading up to the race, I knew that my future wagers on Roadster were in a lot of trouble. I had given out my selections for the Derby on Xpressbet.com, which reaches roughly 20,000 people, a few days before, providing choices for both a fast track and a wet track. There is nothing worse than having to give out my picks two or three days before the race on the radio, TV, and Xpressbet not knowing the weather and, most importantly, how the track is playing on that particular day. There are days that speed horses can't win on the front end and others when it plays in their favor. Every day is different and that's why you have to watch the races on that day to see how the track is playing.

Three weeks before the Derby, Code of Honor caught my eye in his morning workouts. I thought he was sitting on a big race and the price would be right, meaning it was a value play. I loved Code of Honor regardless of what type of track it was and stayed true to my overall picks. Code of Honor was 16-1 in the wagering at post time and Roadster was 11-1. Maximum Security was the second choice at more than 4-1.

I was stationed on the second floor right by the betting windows and the ATMs. If you're going to make your picks, why not do it in an area where people are betting? It was a great decision by our NBC production team. I had a TV monitor and my touchscreen for wagering and teaching purposes. Lots and lots of fans came to our set to say hello and talk pucks and ponies. When I am at the track during the Triple Crown series, people want to talk hockey, and when I am at the rink, people want to talk horses. You gotta love it!

In the fifth race, I liked Hungry Kitten, which was racing for the third time in her career and had not won to that point. She was 12-1 in the morning line and 5-1 at post time, so clearly somebody liked her. I don't know if a lot of that was Edzo money or not because I touted Hungry Kitten on the broadcast. She had a bad post position in her last race but made a nice run. She had blinkers this time and I thought if there was enough speed in the race that jockey Joel Rosario would get the horse out and make a run. I had won the race before with a 6-1 shot, so I was alive in the daily double with two horses in the second leg. But Hungry Kitten was the best play. All the signs were there for her to run well; the question was whether she was good enough to win. Hungry Kitten got up in the final strides to win, so it was nice to get off to a good start on Derby Day after a bad day before.

The video of my reaction to Hungry Kitten's run was very animated. Whether I'm sitting on my couch at home or working, I'm going to try to do what I can to get the horse home if I have a vested interest. It's more than just the financial gains; it's the excitement of finding that horse or horses and coming up with the right combination. I'm hoping to make some money for people watching and betting on my picks.

I had about 25 or 30 texts and I didn't check my phone for a while because I was working. The next thing I know, I've got 300 texts. How the hell do I respond? I need to find that button on my phone with reply all. They all wanted to know who I liked in the Derby and I just planned to reply with the numbers of Tacitus (8), Code of Honor (13), Roadster (17), and Game Winner (16) in various wagers, and Code of Honor to win, place, and show. I was confident Code of Honor would finish in the top three. He was 14-1 at post time. I told one friend to bet all he could on Code of Honor to show, meaning the horse merely needed to finish in the top three of the final order of finish. Depending on the final odds, you are going to cash; it's just a matter of how much.

Like all of NBC's reporters, I was on trainer duty, watching the race from the paddock where the horses are saddled prior to the race. That is where many of the media members are because that's where high-profile trainers such as Bob Baffert and Todd Pletcher watch the race. My assignment was to interview Todd if he won, while at the same time watching the horses I used in my bets.

When Code of Honor was making a move along the rail and briefly had the lead with a quarter of a mile to go, I started to make my way toward Code of Honor's legendary trainer Shug McGaughey, who watches from the owners' and trainers' lounge in the tunnel, which is about 75 yards from the paddock. Once I saw Maximum Security regain the lead, I retreated on tracking down Shug.

Maximum Security, the second choice in the betting at 9-2, seized the lead at the top of the stretch and went on to win by more than 3 lengths over 65-1 long shot Country House. But Maximum Security, ridden by Luis Saez, veered out turning from the two path and into the four or five path going around the final turn into the stretch and impeded some horses in behind.

Watching the race on the big-screen TV in the paddock, I immediately thought there was going to be a stewards' inquiry. My job is to communicate with the production truck if I see something. When Maximum Security veered out, I gave our team a heads-up.

We immediately learned there was a claim of foul by Flavien Prat, the jockey of Country House. The stewards didn't put up the inquiry sign at that point—I have no reason why—and we had no idea that Jon Court, the jockey of Long Range Toddy, had also lodged a claim of foul. That wasn't sent out until a press release was issued two or three hours later. The only info anyone had was that there was one jockey's claim of foul on Maximum Security.

Producer Rob Hyland and director Drew Esocoff did an amazing job of getting all the pictures and interviews that we needed, talking to the right parties and explaining to viewers what was happening. Because we did not get all the information, we had to trust the information we did have, and that's what made it difficult. I thought it would have been a different tone if the stewards had announced there were two jockeys claiming foul.

When I was asked on the broadcast if Country House had been impeded, I said he was, but not much. There was no doubt in my mind that Maximum Security impeded War of Will and Long Range Toddy as well. He also bumped Code of Honor along the rail. There was a lot going on there.

I think the stewards got caught up in the moment. You've got 25 million people watching and almost $390 million bet on the Derby. Country House's trainer Bill Mott said on our broadcast that if this had been a $16,000 maiden claiming race on any other day of the week, the winner would have been taken down right away. He was right, but this was the Derby, so it was a question of whether the stewards would let the history of the Derby influence their decision.

After a 22-minute wait, during which time we repeatedly showed the stewards watching footage of the race from various angles, Maximum Security was disqualified. He became the first winner in the 145-year history of the race to be disqualified and placed 17th in the field of 19 because he was deemed to have interfered with Long Range Toddy, who finished 17th and ended up being placed in behind him in the official running order. Country House was declared the winner, becoming the horse with the second-longest odds to win in race history, paying $132.40 for a $2 ticket.

It took courage on the biggest stage of thoroughbred racing to make that call. Let me make it perfectly clear I agreed with the stewards' decision. How they went about it and how it got there, that's up for debate. But the end result from where I was standing was the right call.

Code of Honor ran third, behind Maximum Security and Country House, and was promoted to second, so I benefitted from the DQ. Code of Honor paid $15.20 to place and $9.80 to show, and I had $400 to place and $600 to show. I had the superfecta once and it paid more than $51,000. I also had the tri once and it paid $11,475.30 for a $2 bet. Overall, I bet about $4,300 on the race. I had a brutal day on Friday, so I broke even for the two days.

Some people think I'm the luckiest guy in the world. No argument here; sometimes you need to make your luck, other times it just happens. Trust me, every horseplayer will tell you there are long stretches of no luck as well. It's like the stock market: you gotta ride the wave. As for betting, there's definitely luck involved and this was another example of beating the odds.

I do believe that if Johnny Velazquez, the rider of Code of Honor, had finished second, he would have claimed foul on the winner. There was enough evidence to show his horse breaking his momentum because of Maximum Security coming back down on the rail and bumping him. Initially, I wasn't looking at that. I was just looking at what was going on in the run around the turn and then watching the replay after the fact.

What I couldn't figure out was, why didn't War of Will's jockey Tyler Gaffalione or trainer Mark Casse claim foul? Their horse finished seventh. Kenny Rice, my NBC colleague, was talking to Mark off camera after the race and asked him what he thought. Mark said after seeing the replay, he probably should have claimed foul as well. Overall, it was very, very lucky no horse or jockey fell to the ground in that race. It was that close to being a disaster, but thank God it wasn't.

There are some people who believe Tyler Gaffalione did not claim foul because the horse kind of forced his way into a hole that wasn't there and started a chain reaction with Maximum Security. So, if Tyler or Mark opened up a can of worms, then maybe the horse would have been disqualified from seventh because he interfered with Long Range Toddy. I can see why team War of Will didn't claim foul, but that was a question many people had. I did not see it that way—this was all on Maximum Security.

On our broadcast, Randy Moss said if there's anybody that's got a beef it's War of Will, specifically Tyler Gaffalione. A jockey's lifeline is owners and trainers. It's about relationships. If a rider lodges a claim of foul, they might lose some business from that owner or trainer because of that. I get it. It's definitely food for thought.

There were many who wondered what made this Derby different from any other Derby that featured a lot of bumping. I always try to consider whether the interference affected the outcome of the race. Nobody can sit there and say Long Range Toddy was going to hit the board. I don't know that for sure. How does anybody know for sure?

I compare what happened in the race to an old hockey phrase: you can clutch and you can grab, but you can't clutch *and* grab. Maximum Security did both of those and that's why he ended up in the penalty box and placed 17th.

In the five years I've been covering the Derby, I've seen two Triple Crowns and the first Derby winner disqualified in 145 years of the race. It's been pretty eventful, that's for sure. Neither the horse that won nor the horse that was promoted to first raced in the Preakness Stakes. This was the first time since 1996 a Derby winner didn't race in the second leg of the Triple Crown.

Two weeks later in Baltimore at the Preakness, I predicted in my Xbressbet pick that Bourbon War was the horse to beat. He had last run fourth in the Florida Derby, so he was fresh, was adding blinkers this time, had a great workout going into the race, would benefit with his closing speed, and had a great starting post. He was a solid 12-1 in the morning line but was bet down to less than 6-1 by post time. The wise guys were on to this horse. War of Will was 4-1 in the morning line, but escalated to more than 6-1. The track was favoring horses on the inside and War of Will was running from the one hole again. When the race began, Bodexpress dumped jockey Johnny Velasquez and ran with the pack. Horses are herd animals and though this had happened countless times before in races all year long, it was something that was a first for the Triple Crown and it attracted a lot of attention. History had been made once again.

War of Will, ridden again by Tyler Gaffalione, won the race by 1¼ lengths over Everfast, who was almost a 30-1 long shot. Mark Casse said it was more a case of his horse having a chance to show what he could do and less about redemption. Bourbon War finished 9½ lengths back in the field of 13.

I cashed on a daily double with War of Will and Catholic Boy in the previous race. The track was playing perfectly for War of Will because the rail was golden on Preakness day. I stuck with Bourbon War, whose only chance was if his jockey Irad Ortiz Jr. kept him on the rail, which he didn't. Even though I picked Bourbon War, I knew he was up against it the way the track was playing kindly to horses on the rail and speed types. I touted War of Will on the broadcast 45 minutes before the race and told Mike Tirico, our NBC host for the Preakness, that War of Will was the "value" play at 6-1. I was shocked his price was that high. Now on any picks I give out on radio, TV, or online, I have to hedge a bit, which I hate doing. But considering I got burned on Preakness day, I have to be able to change my mind before the race depending on how the track is playing. That's handicapping.

Mark Casse had two horses in the Belmont, but it was long shot Sir Winston and not War of Will that won.

A few days later I returned to the hockey booth for the Stanley Cup Final. The St. Louis Blues, who started the new year last overall in the NHL, won the Cup over the Boston Bruins. It was an incredible finish to the Stanley Cup playoffs that saw the four division leaders knocked out in the first round.

I had a little break and then I was off to England to be part of NBC's coverage of the Royal Ascot meet. It was my first time broadcasting (and) betting English races. I was decked out in top hat and tails. What an experience!

Pucks and ponies, you gotta love it.

CHAPTER 24

THANK GOD I GOT SICK

BEING A CANCER SURVIVOR has become front and center in my life. Outside of the kids Diana and I have been blessed with and raised, surviving cancer is probably the greatest achievement in my life—and I've achieved a lot of things. I've had an amazing life and I'm hoping it's not even half over. Considering what cancer is and what I was able to conquer with the help of so many people, I'm lucky to be alive. I've beaten the odds more than once.

During the entire time I was battling cancer, I never once asked, why me? If anything, I was happy it was me, rather than any of the people I truly care about. I would not want anyone I know to go through this. The physical part of it to me was hard, but the toughest battle was the psychological, wondering whether I was going to die, how it was affecting the people around me, and what would happen when the treatments were done. I didn't know if I was going to have to continue the treatments. The toughest part is not knowing.

I'd never thought about suicide in my life, but when I was going through this and taking all this medicine and becoming depressed, it entered my mind. You wonder, is this really worth it? Do I really want to put myself and my family through this? It's sad to say, but there's no doubt the medicine makes you feel that way.

I don't consider myself a religious person, but I do believe in God and prayer and there were probably a handful of times when I communicated with God and asked for help to get me through this battle. I know I had a lot of people praying for me and pulling for me, but I didn't become any more or less religious. I just believed it happened to me for a reason and because I could handle it, even though I didn't know what the end result would be. I'll admit I was scared. I'm not embarrassed to say that.

So many people have asked me if I look at things differently now. For a lot of people, there's a change of priorities when something like this happens. All of a sudden you don't look at things the same. You value things a little bit more. Traffic doesn't bother you. Material things don't matter as much.

Before I got sick, I thought I was in a good place in life, content and at peace with where I was. So, I don't appreciate anything more. But it reassured me I was in a really good place. I was at peace because the most important people in my life knew how I felt about them.

What I also learned is just how difficult it is for some people to talk to someone going through cancer. A lot of people don't know what to say in this type of situation. I understand it's not an easy conversation to have with somebody you love or respect, but in today's world it's easy to communicate with somebody—text, email, Twitter. If you don't reach out to somebody you know in this situation, that makes it worse for them. If somebody means something to you and is going through a cancer battle, or any battle, I would urge you to reach out and say something. It could be as easy as saying, "I'm thinking about you and I'm praying for you."

JOHN McDONOUGH
Blackhawks president and CEO

By him amplifying this for other people to get colonoscopies and maybe creating a little bit of urgency along the way, there was an opportunity to save a lot of lives. He became something of a crusader. If people just read about this for the first time, they would say that's not real. But there are more chapters left. I don't think his story is written yet.

JAY BLUNK
Blackhawks executive vice president

Eddie always felt strongly that his cancer diagnosis and treatment be shared with our entire fan base and the city of Chicago. His purpose of recovering on a public stage, sweeping away any privacy, was to help others. Eddie has allowed his journey to be chronicled in detail in hopes of saving lives. Long before his diagnosis, Eddie was known as a hero for many reasons. After his triumph over cancer, Eddie's mission to save lives has reinforced what we already knew. He is an incredible, passionate, selfless person who has proven there is still hope in the world. A champion in every respect of the word.

In this type of situation, you realize who your friends are, and I'll take that with me the rest of my life. Doesn't matter if you're a general manager of an NHL team, a team's PR person, a mentor, a boss, a coach to my kids. For someone to not pull my kids aside and ask them, "How are you doing?" knowing their father is ill is something I will never get over. I will learn from it, bank it, and when someone asks me for a character assessment of that human, look out. Live and learn. There's no excuse for that or for not reaching out to me or anyone in a similar situation. When people called and said they didn't want to bother me, I told them they weren't bothering me. I needed to talk to somebody. I wanted to hear from somebody. I wanted to communicate with somebody. I want people to know it means a lot when they reach out. It helps someone get through a day because the days are so long.

We all take things for granted, it's just human nature. But as I've gotten older, I've developed more patience and can appreciate everything that has happened. I've had enough quiet time to last me a lifetime, and I thought about a lot of stuff. Contrary to what some people may think, I had a pretty good career. I was a pretty good player. The numbers don't lie. I had a lot of success in the National Hockey League and played 16 seasons. It's hard to play 100 games, let alone 1,000 games. I think back to that stretch when I was one of only seven players in the league with 30 or more goals for five consecutive seasons. That's a hell of a run. I'm probably prouder of what I accomplished as hockey player now than I was before, if that makes any sense. I feel better about my career.

RANDY OLCZYK
Eddie's brother
I wasn't surprised he was able to make something good out of something bad. It's one of those things where you get caught up in your own life and you don't realize what's going on in the rest of the world. People are stricken with cancer and worse all the time. You have to stop and be thankful for what you have. He's the type of guy who was strong enough to get through it and luckily it was contained and he was able to overcome it.

Dealing with cancer will be with me the rest of my life. A tumor popped up out of the blue and suddenly I had Stage 3 colon cancer. So anytime I go back to the hospital or have a checkup, I'm always apprehensive and hope everything is okay. Prior to my cancer diagnosis, I never worried about going to the doctor, but now my heart rate goes up. I know I had cancer and beat it and hope the positive news continues.

I know the impact I've had on people by bringing awareness to cancer and, in particular, colon cancer. Mary Higgins, whose husband, Brian, is the director of team security for the Hawks, had a colonoscopy when I became sick and it was discovered she had Stage 3 colon cancer, similar to mine. What happened to her hit so close to home. You talk about salt of the earth people? You're not going to find greater people than Brian and Mary.

BRIAN HIGGINS
Blackhawks director of security

When Eddie recommended everyone get screened, my wife, Mary, got checked. Within about five minutes of Mary being diagnosed with colon cancer, I called Eddie. I believe it was his son's wedding day, which I didn't even realize, and he took the time to talk to us, which is the kind of guy that he is. He and his wife, Diana, sent a nice care package to our house of gifts and things to make Mary comfortable. Eddie's lighting a fire under us may ultimately save her. She probably would have waited a little longer and then it could have become a disaster. God's on our side and so is Eddie.

TROY MURRAY
Eddie's teammate

He's made a lot of people realize that if it can happen to someone like him—a non-smoker and non-drinker—it can happen to anybody. Because of him I had a colonoscopy and was diagnosed with a condition called Barrett's syndrome, which can lead to esophageal cancer. I wouldn't have found that out without Eddie going public.

He's always been a very emotional and passionate person. I think that makes him more relatable to people. They can see the emotion when he talks about what he's gone through and how hard it was for him to even tell his family because he thought he had let them down.

He's not driven by money, fame, or fortune, but I think he understands he is in a position to help others and I think he's done a phenomenal job. I'm proud of him and proud to call him my friend.

I just want people to look after themselves and be proactive, so they won't have to go through what I did. I hope that somebody hears my story and has gotten checked because they weren't feeling good. I feel for people who are going through cancer and want to be there for them if I can help in any way.

I was scheduled to have a colonoscopy in November of that year, so presumably the doctors would have found it then. But if I hadn't gone in with stomach pains four months earlier, who knows what that tumor could have done? If it had spread to my stomach, forget it, just count the days.

Shit happens for a reason—and sometimes it's a good reason—so I thank God I got sick.

AFTERWORD

Throughout this book, I've tried to make it clear how much I relied on my family to get me through this battle with cancer. It was truly a family achievement. It only feels right to give my kids a chance to tell their stories.

EDDIE

On August 6, 2017, my future in-laws, Chris and Kristie Bozin, hosted an engagement party for me and my fiancée, Erika, who is now my wife, at a posh steakhouse in Chicago. The party included 60 family members and guests, but noticeably absent was my dad, Eddie. He found out two days before the engagement party he had Stage 3 colon cancer and would have to undergo chemotherapy treatment. Physically, mentally, and emotionally, my father was in no shape to attend the engagement party. So, while it was a time to rejoice, it was also a time to be concerned.

And not only was it my engagement party, it was also my parents' 29th wedding anniversary.

Though it hurt emotionally not having him there, I didn't resent him for that. It was not his fault. It was a big point of my life and I wanted everybody who mattered to me there to share in that moment. To have it in Chicago and not have him there was really tough. There was a part of me that was experiencing my own joy and taking another step in my life, but also thinking, man, I really wish my dad was here and I wonder if he's going to be okay.

My father was lying in bed with my mother by his side when he received the sobering news he had cancer. Five days before that, he underwent emergency surgery to remove a tumor and some lymph nodes. He was told he might have colon cancer, but that wouldn't be confirmed until the results from a biopsy came back. My brothers, Tommy and Nicky, and my sister, Zandra, and I, were downstairs and he and my mother came down from their room to deliver the news. Initial shock set in among us, along with a bunch of questions: Was he going to be okay? Is he going to make it? How bad is it? He answered those questions and said the doctors had a game plan.

When you hear "cancer," you never really know. You think worst-case scenario right away. We were shocked. We were scared. Here's a guy who's never smoked or drank and was in excellent physical condition. He was our hero, our role model, somebody we've always looked up to. Looking back on it, I never thought something like that would be possible. Not for my father.

While shocked, upset, and worried, we just had to put trust in the system and the people caring for him. That is how I internalized it. The chips find a way to fall a lot of different ways when you least expect it.

My concern was how I could be there for my father and mother when it was physically impossible. As an assistant hockey coach at Bemidji State University in Minnesota, I had to leave to prepare for another season. This was emotionally hard for me. With my dad sick and slated to begin treatment, I felt somewhat helpless. I knew that the majority of my communication was going to be on the phone or via text, but I would be there for him. We were all going to be there for him as a family because we are really tight-knit.

When I was talking to him on the phone when he first began chemo, you could hear how tired he was. Conversations weren't like they used to be because his energy level was down. It sounded like he just got up from a nap, like he was kind of groggy. When I asked how he was doing, he said, "I'm doing okay." I think he wanted to be strong because he didn't want us to worry. In conversations with my mother, she said he was struggling. I don't think I really knew how much he was struggling until I talked to my mom.

It was difficult talking to him because I knew he was putting on a little bit of a front. He wanted me and my siblings to know everything was going to be okay. But was it?

As a family, we'd never been through anything like this, and being far away made it impossible to see how he was doing on a day-to-day basis. I had an idea, but I didn't really know, if that makes sense. I could only imagine.

I was able to get back home for Thanksgiving. Our team had a road trip to Princeton and typically I don't go on the road with the team on weekends, because that's when I scout junior teams in one of my primary roles as the recruiting coordinator. I'm watching a ton of hockey every weekend, but my boss, head coach Tom Serratore, told me to go home and be with my family for Thanksgiving. For that, I was very thankful.

This was my first time seeing my dad since he began chemotherapy. It was shocking seeing him like that for the first time, hooked up to a pump and knowing what that medicine was, how it was making him feel. He had gained some weight because of prescribed steroids to help keep up his energy level. He's a fit guy, sweating on the bike every single morning. He was an athlete and that's something that never leaves you— that work ethic and that comfort of having a routine. I think for him it was really depleting to not be able to do what he's always done. Athletes are creatures of habit. Seeing him sluggish and with that added weight really opened my eyes.

My parents sent out a media release through the Chicago Blackhawks indicating my father had colon cancer, that he would be undergoing treatment, and asked for people to respect our privacy. I tweeted something to indicate it had been a very emotional number of days for my family and to thank everyone for the support we received. I wrote that my father is the strongest person I know and he was going to beat cancer. I said he's going to go pound for pound with cancer and be standing with his hands in the air at the end, same as he did scoring 361 times in his career. I received an amazing amount of response and it felt great to know the impact my father had and that so many people were praying for him.

It was really tough at times going into rinks, because the first question people asked was, "How's your dad?" Being the son of a high-profile hockey/horse racing broadcaster, it wasn't like you could hide to get away from the attention. It was something as a family we couldn't really escape.

The good thing was, those people asking were people we knew through the hockey world. I guess it was kind of a blessing in disguise. The hockey world is small, but it's the greatest world because of the relationships that are formed.

It seemed like my dad's name was always popping up through interviews he did for TV, radio, and newspapers. There was considerable interest from the hockey and the horse racing worlds. There was an interview on one of the Canadian sports channels that he did in which he was really emotional. I had some friends text me links to it and it was painful to watch.

When he was cancer-free, he texted us. I remember watching the Hawks game that night in which Pat Foley, my dad's broadcast partner and close friend, interviewed him to tell everyone the good news. I'm a hockey junkie and I was watching it with Erika, and it was kind of cathartic. It was emotional. If anybody was going to beat cancer, it was going to be him. And he did.

Honestly, it was amazing, that's really the best way to describe the feeling. A big weight comes off your shoulders as a family. You're emotionally sad, but happy. You know that he had to go through that struggle, but the fact that he overcame it and persevered made us all feel overjoyed. You see, this wasn't something he battled alone. We were all there for him. As my dad said so often in interviews during the six-month battle, it was a team effort.

He wanted to be well enough to attend our wedding. It was something he jotted down on his calendar as one of his goals. The fact that he was able to make it to the wedding and beat cancer meant so much. The wedding happened on August 4, a year to the day he found out he had cancer. Because of my hectic schedule, we only had two possible dates, so we chose that one. How ironic that it would be the same date my father was told he had colon cancer.

Getting married is a big enough deal as it is, but to have my dad there really made it that much more special. One hundred percent. When you think about your wedding day and all the family and the people who are closest to you there to celebrate it, the first people you think of are your parents. During that whole year leading up to the wedding, I was thinking, what if something were to go wrong and he won't be there for it? It would have been really overwhelming and conflicting to get married without your father there.

I couldn't wait for the toast he would make at the wedding. He touched a lot of hearts, letting people know that there's so much to be thankful for and not to take any day for granted. Live in the now and appreciate what you have. He knocked it out of the park with his words. When he gave that speech it was kind of the climax of the wedding, at least for me. He did a great job and right there it was time for me and for everybody to breathe a sigh of relief and hope we could finally put this in the past.

What I learned through the whole process reiterated everything I already knew about him. He's a blue-collar guy. He's an extremely hard worker, based on how he was raised. My paternal grandfather came over in a boat from Europe, starting out in a grocery store and eventually building his own franchise, having his brothers and my grandma working with him. My grandparents built a life for themselves and their family.

Being a kid from Chicago at a time when hockey wasn't appreciated the way it is now, my dad pursued his passion. But it wouldn't have happened without the support he had from his parents. It's the same support he and my mother have provided for me and my two brothers and sister.

I can honestly say there were many times throughout his cancer battle that I wondered if he would successfully beat it. But I also knew my dad is a fighter, a battler. He worked so hard for everything he has accomplished in his various careers. There's a reason he's one of the most well-known names in all of hockey and horse racing broadcasting. He worked hard for that. Nothing was handed to him. He had to earn it.

Above all he's my dad and I love him and am so thankful he could be at my wedding, healthy and happy. He is blessed. We are all blessed as a family.

My dad is sure it wasn't always easy for me having the same name as him. But I wouldn't have it any other way.

I love you, Dad, and I am so proud to be named Eddie Olczyk.

TOMMY

Obviously, all of my siblings and I have different takes on everything that happened with my dad. Everyone has their own point of view, everyone has their own feelings. We're all related and super close; growing up the way we did cemented that. But at the same time, we're all different people and everyone reacts to tragedy differently.

And that's what it was: a tragedy. The second-strongest person we've ever known (Mom is number one!) got diagnosed with Stage 3 colon cancer.

My little brother Nick and I were fishing in Columbus, Indiana, early in the morning when my dad called. We had just caught a bass and decided to send a picture to him. He didn't come with us because he was scheduled to broadcast a horse race in New Jersey and then decided to skip that because he wasn't feeling well. Now he was telling us we needed to come home because he was in the hospital and in rough shape.

An hour later we were in the car driving to the hospital. At that point we had no idea what his diagnosis was. We just knew he had to undergo some procedures so they could figure it out and fix whatever the issue was.

Eventually we find out there's some sort of mass in my dad's colon that needs to be taken out. He came home a day later and we were all waiting to hear back from the doctors about the results of a biopsy.

A few nights later the phone rang and my parents were upstairs in their room and answered the phone. Then my parents came down and broke the news to us. The mass they removed from my dad was indeed cancerous, and the doctors strongly recommended chemo. It really wasn't even a choice. He had to battle. He had to fight. He had to win. Just like he has his entire life. And he didn't even do it for himself. He did it for my mom—his rock—his parents, his brothers, me and my brothers and sister, and our black Labs, Lily and Daisy. He also fought for the hockey community and all his fans and former teammates. He was battling and fighting for a lot of people and a lot of reasons.

Seeing my dad after his first chemo treatment was horrifying. I was the only one of my siblings who was home for that. I honestly don't even know if Eddie, Nick, or Zandra ever saw that side of my dad. You'd have to ask them. I just know that they weren't there for the first treatment. And that's not a knock on them. Nick and Zandra were in school and Eddie was in Minnesota with his fiancée, Erika, working as the assistant coach of the Bemidji State University hockey team. It's not like they didn't want to be there. I was just the one caught between college and the real world. I played minor pro hockey because I could—and it beats a real job—so I was home throughout.

So, I was there for the first one. It was the first time I ever had to give my father a pep talk.

"I don't think I can do this, Thomas," he said.

Those were his first words to me the first time he got sick. Now, I'm not a very emotional person and empathy is not one of my best qualities, but to be honest, in that situation it probably worked in my favor.

"I don't care, Dad. Toughen up. You don't have a choice," I said.

That's a super insensitive thing to say, I'm not naive, but I truly believe he needed to hear that. He didn't have a choice. He had to fight. He had to survive. And he did.

Personally, I felt a little guilty that year. I was home during his first round of chemo. I wanted to be home to take care of him. To kick him in the butt when he needed it. To make him laugh by quoting the Austin Powers movies. To just be there for him like he has always been there for me.

But he didn't want that. He didn't need that. He knew we were there to support him, even if we were hundreds of miles away. The best medicine for him was knowing that all of his children were off following their dreams, doing what made them happy.

And what drove him throughout his battle was wanting to be there for all of our future accomplishments. And he will be.

He was there for Eddie's wedding. He'll be there for mine. He'll be around when Nick graduates college in a couple of years. And he'll be there to walk my sister down the aisle one day. Why? Because he's a warrior. He's a fighter. He was never the strongest hockey player. He was never the fastest or the most feared. But when it comes to life, he is the toughest and hardest-working person I know.

He's my hero.

ZANDRA

I was getting ready to go on a date when I heard my phone ring. It was my mom. I had been at the University of Alabama for summer school and for some reason that whole day I felt off and I couldn't pinpoint why. When I saw it was her calling, I just knew something was wrong.

I answered and she said Dad was in the hospital. I felt sick, the kind of sick you feel that can bring you to your knees. The doctors weren't sure what was going on but they were doing all they could to figure it out. I knew Dad was not feeling well days leading up to this, but we thought it was kidney stones, something he's had several times before. I knew in my gut this was different. I was so upset and felt helpless because there was nothing anyone could do.

After my mom and I talked, I spoke with my dad and tried to hold back the tears because I didn't want to make him more upset and scared. I told him I loved him and it would be okay; he was where he needed to be and they would figure it out. He reassured me he was okay (typical Dad) and not to worry and to focus on my summer courses. My dad's a tough guy, anyone could tell you that, but even though he was comforting me, I knew he was scared and that worried me.

I had to go home. I couldn't sleep that night, tossing and turning, unsure of what was to come. But somehow, I knew he would be okay. He had the best care, people, and family looking after him.

The following day, I cleared things up with my professors and rearranged my class schedule so I could hop on a flight to be with him and my family. To me that's what was and is most important.

My three brothers, my mom, and I were sitting around the table having a family dinner. We hadn't had one in ages due to being scattered all over the place, whether it was due to work or school. It was so nice to finally be with each other again at home, but given the circumstances things were different and something was missing at dinner: Dad. He wasn't feeling well, so he skipped dinner and stayed in bed.

Waiting for that phone call after the biopsy, every sound that we heard, whether it was the scratching of forks against our plates or random TV sounds, made us jumpy and edgy. Mom went to check on Dad to see if he needed anything. Time passed; it felt like hours. Mindless eating and limited conversation.

Finally, the house phone rang. We get random calls all the time, but we all just knew this was *the* call.

Everyone stopped, shared uneasy glances, and waited for Mom and Dad to come downstairs. They took a little too long. I felt my heart racing and beating through my chest while I was going back and forth in my mind. I was hoping they hadn't come down yet because they were celebrating good news. But what if something really was wrong?

We heard their hard and heavy footsteps coming down each stair, which rocked each of us to our cores. I just knew something was off. Dad was visibly shaken, but kept his composure while slowly walking over to the table. At that moment, we knew. Mom and Dad reached the head of the table and told us he had cancer. Each of us dropped our heads and just blankly stared at the table.

I'm a very sensitive and emotional person, but I didn't know how to feel in that moment, which shocked me. I felt numb from head to toe. I prefer to be emotional in private because I don't want to make anyone more upset than they are. But I was angry. I just wanted to scream at the top of my lungs and cry, but I knew we had to be strong for him because that's what families do. You are always there for one another no matter what happens. My dad has always been strong for us and I knew this is the time we had to be strong for him.

This was one of those awful moments in life that you never think will happen to you—or at least, you hope they don't. When it does, you almost go into a fog and shock where you're not sure what is happening. I was blank. I tried to keep it all in. I didn't want my dad getting more upset, but what really got me was seeing my brothers cry and how affected they were, which made me start to cry. We hugged my dad and told him it was all going to be okay. We wouldn't let it not be okay. That day was a beyond brutal day, but he got through it like we knew he would because that's who he is, a fighter.

My mom held my dad's hand and said we would get through this as a family. She said it would be hard on all of us, but we had to be there for one another no matter what and to check in on each other and on Dad. She said to remember that we get through these things together, like we've done everything else.

Hearing my mom say everything would be all right, being the rock that she is, just empowered us all to know we would fight this with him.

Something deep down inside me knew things would be okay. Knowing who my dad is and his true spirit showed clearly that things would be okay, even if it didn't look like it on the surface. Being away from home during this time was hard—*really* hard. Like I mentioned, I'm a sensitive person and once I get hooked on thinking about something that means a lot to me, I can't stop. I get fixated.

While I was away at college, all I cared about was how my dad was doing. I put on a brave face and covered up how I was really doing. No one knew because I felt selfish. I didn't go to classes. I laid in bed or I went out. I felt guilty being so far from home and going to college where you're told to "have fun." How could I when my dad was going through this? I kept thinking how healthy he was—he's a professional athlete, for gosh sakes. You wake up one day and everything changes.

After a few weeks of this downward spiral, I knew I had to change and to be strong for him, but it didn't seem to get easier. I wasn't sure why. I was told all the treatments were going well and he was doing great, but I was just still so mad. I didn't want to be at school. I wanted to be home because my mind was wandering and I wasn't sure what was going to happen. I wanted to be spending those crucial moments with him and helping my mom. There was so much put on the both of them. I wanted to help. But they told me I was helping by doing well in school and graduating in the fall. They said, "Your place is at school. You need to live your life. That's what we want for you and what makes us happy as your parents." That finally woke me up. It wasn't about me: it was about Dad, and what he needed from me was to do well and focus on my future.

During this time, I was lucky enough to have amazing friends in college and from home who were my support, as well as my amazing brothers. We always checked up on each other and vented when we needed to. It wasn't easy but we got through it because we had to for Dad. Mindset is everything and when it's not good, life goes terribly wrong. There had to be a mental change for me and I found that in my classes, friends, and family. You realize how grateful you are for your family when you go through things like this. I knew I had to do well for him because he wanted to be here to see me graduate, and that's what I did.

Graduation came in December and meant a lot to me, even more than any other thing I've done (which hasn't been a lot, ha ha). Being able to look up in the stands after walking across the stage (and not falling may I add, which was an accomplishment in itself) and seeing my mom and dad waving at me and screaming my name meant so much. It was not only an accomplishment on my end, but for him as well. He kept saying he wanted to be there, and he was. It brought tears to my eyes, not because I had just graduated but because he was able to be there. He did what he set his mind to for me. It meant so much. He's never missed a big moment in my life and he certainly didn't that day. He probably felt horrible and wanted to be in bed, but he didn't show it and was such a proud father that day, which made me bawl. I'm so lucky to have shared that day with my parents. It will always be one of my happiest memories.

My mom and dad are just special humans. They are great people and even better parents. Even through all the changes in life they made it clear that we were their priority. They love us and would do anything for us because they care so deeply, and that always showed and always will. We've always been a close family. Moving all over the place throughout the years will do that to you. You change schools, friends, and places so often that having your siblings around and to call them your friends is really special. Not everyone has that. Just because you are family doesn't mean you have to like each other, but I genuinely can say that's not the case for us. From my earliest memories, we always did things as a family and were truly happy. It brings a smile to my face. We were and are always supportive of one another. Whether it was traveling to cheer each other on in sports, family vacations, or just funny memories, we always had each other. Sure, we've had our issues over the years, who hasn't? But I'm so lucky to have them in my life. I love my friends, but no one will come close to my family. Any way we could, no matter the distance, we were there for each other.

You don't realize how much hard times change you as a family until you're going through it. This made us closer and stronger. We did what we always do when anything comes up for us as a family—we got through it together.

They say God gives his greatest challenges to those who can handle them, even if it doesn't feel like that sometimes. But I truly believe in that, especially after all my dad went though. He's one of the strongest people I know. With the platform he has, he is able to help others and bring awareness to this disease. The outpouring of love and support just showed who he is as a person—a great soul. He's a true hero to many. He has helped change lives, including his own.

My dad's always been a funny and energetic guy and I feel that is even more true after this battle. It gave him a new perspective. He has always been there for us, as well as for people he doesn't know. He never says "no." He never missed a dance recital of mine. He was always a present parent and I'll always be so thankful for that. He goes above and beyond and I'm so grateful to have him around. I'm thankful for all the memories we have and are going to have in the future.

Having dad and daughter breakfast and lunch dates growing up, driving me to school, blaring music and embarrassing me, shopping for Mom at Christmas, those are the memories that make me smile and remind me how great of a dad he is. Hearing people say great things about him and saying I am lucky to have him as my dad, well, I already knew that to be true. But he's my father and growing up you just say, "Oh, well, that's just my dad."

As I've gotten older and everything that had happened over the last year, I've realized how true that all is. He's just the best. Who doesn't go through phases of thinking their parents are bothering them or are uncool? But I'm beyond lucky to have him as my dad.

Anytime I've ever needed advice or just to talk, no matter what he was doing, he was there for me. He may not have been physically around much due to work, but he always made it clear he loves us and is proud to be our dad. Well, I'm proud of him and I love him.

I say my dad is "one" of the strongest people I know, because my mom is the other one. She was his rock during this grueling time period. This really opened my eyes to how amazing their love and respect is for one another. My mom is the definition of a tough cookie. She doesn't take anything from anyone, but is also the kindest and most generous person I've ever known. The journey was the furthest thing from easy, but Mom helped open my dad's eyes to see he had to fight for all of us, even when he felt he couldn't do it anymore. My dad is headstrong and seeing he was losing that during this time was beyond difficult. No one knew what to do because no one can ever prepare you for how mentally exhausting this could be. He got through it, even when he didn't think he could, and the biggest reason was my mom.

They complement one another and help each other when one is down, and in this case, it was him. It makes me realize I won't settle for anyone who doesn't respect, love, and care for me like my parents do for each other.

This was a hard time but it helped them grow even closer together, which I didn't think could happen after 30 years of marriage. Once again, I'm in awe of them. I'm lucky to have them both in my life and am so thankful they have shown us how a true marriage should be, no matter what—in sickness and in health.

NICK

We were there with my dad in his hospital room before he underwent the surgery. When the nurse came in and said the doctors were ready to go, my mom embraced him and gave him a kiss and Grandpa did the same. As they left the room I kind of hung back and looked at my dad. He looked back at me and we both started bawling. I get choked up just thinking about it.

I'd never, ever seen him cry before. Superman doesn't cry. That was really the first time I ever saw my dad get emotional. I walked over to him and placed my head on his chest and tried to grip him as hard as I could. He embraced me in the very same fashion, squeezing my head and my body and saying, "It's going to be okay." That's a moment that is burned into my memory. When I look back on this battle, that is the one image and scene that keeps coming back—me pressed against his chest and not wanting to let him go as the nurse in the background said, "Are you ready to go, Mr. Olczyk?"

I've had friends whose family members have been diagnosed with cancer, but when it's someone else you say, "I feel bad." But it doesn't really rock you to the core. When that happened to my dad, it took a whole other turn. My dad is everything you could want in a father. When you hear that word and it applies to your own father, you think, maybe he's not going to be around and maybe he is not Superman. That's certainly scary.

I was set to leave for my freshman year at Colorado College two weeks later. I was on a partial hockey scholarship but I wanted to stay home. I wanted to be here and take care of my dad because he took care of me for the last 22 years. Yeah, I knew my mom was home, my grandparents were at home, and my sister would be around as well, but being his son, I thought it was my duty to wait on him hand and foot. That's just what I thought the responsibility was as a son, just as he has had a responsibility as a father for me and my brothers and sister and continues to do that to this day. Love is unconditional and unlimited.

I was prepared to take a gap year, stay at home, and do whatever I could to help. If it had to be a break in my hockey and school career, then so be it. Nothing is more important than family.

After my parents told us he had cancer, I followed him back up to his room and kind of shut the door. With tears in my eyes and my hands and feet shaking, I said, "Dad, I can't go to school. I'm not going to leave you here. I know there are other people here, but it's too big of a weight for me to leave."

He looked back at me and kind of grabbed me and said, "Look, you only would be hurting me more if you stay. I don't want to be the reason for you to have to put your life on hold or sacrifice anything."

When he told me that, something changed in me. I was still upset and I still wanted to stay, but I kind of understood what he was saying. That was a brave thing for him to say and I wouldn't have expected anything less, but it was hard. I didn't really accept that answer because I was so emotionally drained and still emotionally hyped up in the same moment. I wanted to be there for him and he wanted me to go to school, so it was a mix of emotions. Again, I'd like to make clear that I was prepared to stay and that's what I had my heart set on.

Once I left their bedroom, I practically sprinted to mine. I sat down on my bed with my hands on my face, trying to hold back the tears. Being someone who is open and social, my first moves were to call those I loved and tell them the news. My first two calls were to my girlfriend at the time, Carley, as well as my best friend since I was nine-years-old, Joey. I was choked up while telling him the news and he became extremely emotional as well. I had never heard him cry either. This was a powerful moment between us because we had been playing hockey together since we were in the fourth grade, and our families had been tied together ever since. Seeing the effect this news had on my friends helped me gain perspective and realize the magnitude that my father's situation had on so many other people than just me and my immediate family.

Leaving to go to school was extremely difficult. I had this cloud of guilt hanging over me, despite my dad telling me I had to go and do what's best for me. I still felt deep down I should be at home.

News of my father's illness shook the hockey and the horse racing worlds. I received calls, texts, and Twitter messages from both people I knew and didn't know, telling me to send their wishes his way. Things like that meant a lot and just went to show that this world will always come together when people need other people the most; I can speak to that firsthand.

There were times that I called him and the conversation would be kind of short and I could tell he was hurting. All I wanted to do was be there for him, whether to pick him up some lunch or to tell him a joke and see him smile. I felt guilty for not being a physical presence. I talk to my parents every day. We're extremely close and there's not a day that goes by that I don't speak to both of them. But in this case, it got to a point where maybe I was calling my dad too much. I remember a specific phone call, the second or third call I made to him one day, and he said, "Nick, I'm fine. You don't have to keep calling. We do our daily phone call and you don't have to do it more."

There were those late moments at night where I would sit there and wonder if he was going to be there tomorrow or next week or next year. Coming to grips with that was by far the toughest thing I've ever had to face in my life. Harder than any hockey game. Harder than any rep in the gym. Harder than any test I've ever had to take in school. The idea that he might pass and no longer be a presence in my life was a devastating thought, but I also had a reason to be optimistic knowing the battler that he is and how strong he is mentally and physically.

I came home for Thanksgiving, which was rare because usually there's a Thanksgiving hockey tournament. Our team did not have one, so I was finally able to see my dad for the first time since I had left for school. The effects from the chemo most certainly took their toll on him and the way he looked, but he was still my dad and I loved him, whether he was

40 pounds overweight or 40 pounds underweight. As a guy who works out religiously and does his cardio bike every single morning, this was a struggle for him. The steroids never allowed his stomach to be satisfied, so the tendency became to eat and eat and then eat some more.

I returned for Christmas, which is always special for us because we're a close family and have had a lot of great Christmases. We love the holidays. Having four kids so spread out and my dad consistently being on the road doing games made us savor those moments and really appreciate the time we have together.

We host Christmas Eve dinner at our house with my uncles and cousins. What I remember most about this Christmas Eve was my mom saying the prayer that night—I'm getting a little emotional just thinking about it. She said, "Please, God, watch over us and keep those who have been affected by illness in your thoughts."

I couldn't help but look up and take a peek at my dad. It was one of the very few times that I saw him get teary-eyed. As tears fell from his eyes they began to fall from mine, and I quickly looked back down because I didn't want to show any kind of sadness. We had to be positive and strong for him.

There were times over the Christmas break when my dad was nearly unable to move from the couch and needed me to get him a glass of water with a lemon—and easy on the ice, of course. Once we were both sitting on the couch in the basement watching hockey. He was cold and reached for a pair of socks. Attempting to put them on himself, he struggled mightily. In this moment, watching out of the corner of my eye, I saw the struggle going on within his mind and in his body. He looked at me dead in the eye and asked if I would help.

Jumping at the opportunity to be of assistance, I reached for the socks and slid them on his feet. When he said, "Thank you, Nick," I could feel a sense of embarrassment in my father. As the prideful man that he is, he still understood that it's necessary to ask for help in times of need, and there wasn't a single moment in which I wasn't ready to help. Though it was a small request, in that moment he overcame his pride and asked for help. If there's one thing that hockey players and horseplayers have in common, it's that they are both full of pride and a sense of independence. But if I've learned anything from my dad during his battle, it's that when things don't feel right, ask for a helping hand. There's no shame in doing so, because at one point or another we all need the assistance of others.

Each plane ride I took back to school, I felt more and more comfortable with the situation. My dad's positivity and reassurances helped in a massive way. At the end of the day, positivity always wins out.

I will never forget the day my dad told me he was cancer-free. I was still at school and coming back from lunch. When I answered my phone, I heard a tone in his voice that I hadn't heard in a long time. I didn't know if he had hit a Pick 6 or won the lottery. It wasn't an exuberant, "Hey, Nick, how's it going?" It was more like, "Hey, Nick." I stopped in my tracks and said, "Is everything okay? Did we win the lottery?" We kind of had.

He said, "Nick, I'm clean now."

I had my left hand holding the phone to my ear and did a huge fist pump with my right hand. I'm sure the three people who walked by me thought I was crazy, but I celebrated as if I had just scored a goal. As a family, that's kind of what we did. We went through the other team's whole defense and made a beautiful backhand move around the goaltender and scored.

There aren't many moments that bring you to your knees, but that one really did because it was a total release. Through all the struggles, the heartache, and the guilt I felt, he was clean now. It was a huge weight off our shoulders. I've had a lot of good phone calls in my life, but that was the best I ever received.

So, what did I learn about my dad through all of this? Well, I've always thought of my dad as Superman, someone who is strong and had a vision and knew exactly what he wanted to do. He had all those prototypical superhero attributes. He is determined and brave and stuck to his convictions. I've learned a thousand life lessons from him over the course of my life, and what I learned throughout his cancer battle is he is exactly the man that he appears to be. When you hear him, when you see him, when you talk to him, he really is that genuine as a person. I can sit here and say he beat cancer, so he is strong and brave and courageous. But he was all that stuff before cancer. It's a battle that can deteriorate you and leave you in complete oblivion if you let it. He was positive about it.

I remember the TV interview he did with David Kaplan, who is a prominent sports broadcaster in Chicago and one of my dad's closest friends. He was asked about the illness and his kids and he said, "I'm glad it was me." That is the ultimate father comment there. He added that if it had happened to any of us, he didn't know what he would do. That speaks to the character that he has and the type of man that he is.

With everything he is doing now to raise awareness about colon cancer and telling people to get checked out, it's amazing. The easy thing to do when you're in the public eye and going through a battle like that is to feed off of the so-called publicity and all the well-wishes, and then not do anything with that opportunity once you beat it. He has gone to great lengths to speak about it and done countless interviews. To him, if he can help a person avoid going through what he did, it was all worth it.

Especially once I left home at 17 to pursue my aspirations playing junior hockey, my dad wasn't able to see many of my games in person. His heavy workload and travel schedule meant he watched the majority of my games on his computer. He'd sometimes watch my games out of the corner of his eye while broadcasting his games. That is truly remarkable and something that I'll forever appreciate and be grateful for. He's the ultimate hockey parent: knowledgeable, demanding, understanding, compassionate, and most of all willing to teach the greatest game in the world. His mixture of hard love and constant reminders to be your best all the time, not just half of the time, are lessons that I'll carry with me for the rest of my life.

He is the man that I strive to be every day. He really is Superman.

ACKNOWLEDGMENTS

THERE ARE SO MANY thank-yous to pass around on my journey to this point in my life. All of this started at home with the original Ed and Diana, my folks. They taught my brothers, Ricky and Randy, and I the value of loyalty, discipline, and the power of belief. We were given support, guidance, and a lot of love that still exists to this day.

The game of hockey has opened up thousands of relationships and doors for me, one of them being horse racing, beginning at age 12 through the father of a teammate. Pucks and ponies, nothing better! Through the two sports I have developed so many friends who are like family.

I am grateful to all of the teams I played for, teammates, coaches, front office staff, trainers, broadcast partners, TV production crews, and fans. It truly has been tremendously tremendous.

A big thank-you to all the people who have helped with this book, especially Perry Lefko, who had this idea a long time ago and eventually opened my eyes to how I could share my story and maybe help someone out there as well.

I played a long time in the National Hockey League, scored a few goals, and played in some great cities along the way, but I believe my greatest accomplishment is my family: my wife, Diana, who is the rock in our family, and our four kids, Eddie, Thomas, Alexandra, and Nick.

There have been plenty of obstacles and potholes along the way. Life is not easy. I would give anything to go back 15 years, not to do more or provide more, but to have more time with them. It has gone by way too fast. They have made my life complete I am so proud and thankful for them.

They are my life! Life is family!

—Eddie Olczyk

I FIRST MET EDDIE Olczyk back in the early 1990s when I was reporting on horse racing for the *Toronto Sun*. He and teammate Gary Leeman owned thoroughbred horses and I wrote some stories about that.

I also made some bets for Eddie when he wanted to make some wagers at Woodbine Racetrack but was on the road with the Leafs. He left me money and I'd call him up wherever his horses were running, held up the phone to the TV, and let him listen.

I lost contact with Eddie as our paths went separate ways, but I reconnected with him shortly after he was diagnosed with Stage 3 colon cancer. I reached out to him to wish him well and also to ask if I could interview him for the *Thoroughbred Daily News*. He agreed and I followed that up with more articles during his journey.

I then approached him about the idea of working together on a book about his life and career, principally his cancer battle and how he handled it. We had talked about doing a book a few years earlier but it didn't go anywhere, likely because the timing wasn't right or maybe there needed to be an impetus to do it. His successful battle with cancer and how he spoke about it publicly with passion and honesty provided that impetus.

We began working on the book and Eddie did not hesitate to discuss sensitive subjects. It wasn't all doom and gloom, however. When we talked about horse racing and some of his scores, Eddie really perked up. On several occasions when we got together either at his home or various other places, horse racing was on the TV or a screen nearby. Sometimes in the middle of a conversation, he paused to watch a race before continuing his train of thought.

This project would not have happened without Eddie's help. He believed in my vision for this and for that I am grateful.

Behind many great hockey players/broadcasters/horseplayers is a great partner, and in Eddie's case it's Diana. I hadn't seen her in almost 30 years, but when we started this project it was as if we had just seen one another. Her insights and suggestions really helped add some context to the overall story.

Eddie and Diana's children—Eddie, Tommy, Alexandra (Zandra), and Nick—helped immensely by explaining how they were individually affected by their father's illness.

Eddie's mother and father, Ed and Diana, opened up their home and their hearts to me. Thanks to Mrs. O for the great licorice cheesecake.

Eddie's brothers, Ricky and Randy, helped with valuable recollections.

I am indebted to all of the people at Triumph Books, especially Noah Amstadter, who embraced this project when I presented it to him, and Adam Motin, who oversaw the editing.

Chicago Blackhawks team physician Dr. Michael Terry provided key medical details about Eddie's surgery and follow-up material.

Dave Fischer of USA Hockey provided names and contact information for various people. Same goes for Josh Rimer, Mike Zeisberger, Lance Hornby, Bob Irving, Rob Vanstone, and Judy Owen, who collectively have a great list of contacts.

Jim Cressman, one of my journalism mentors, put me in touch with Eddie's Stratford coach, Dave Cressman.

Doug Molleken put me in touch with his brother, Lorne.

Craig Campbell of the Hockey Hall of Fame gave me access to files and articles about Eddie's career.

Carly Napier of the National Hockey League Alumni Association sourced photos.

Kevin Shea, an all-around great hockey writer, gave me key information and support.

Neil Milbert's stories in *The Hockey News* helped immensely. Whether it's hockey or horse racing, Neil's writing is always on point.

Karen Milner and Arnold Gosewich gave me publishing advice.

A special thanks to Chicago Blackhawks president John McDonough and Hawks executive vice president Jay Blunk for their valuable contributions and keen insights about Eddie.

Thanks also to Breeders' Cup chairman Fred Hertrich III and Woodbine Entertainment Group CEO Jim Lawson for their interest in supporting the book.

Eddie's broadcasting "teammate" Pat Foley did an amazing job writing the foreword, and thanks to the great Bob Verdi for his help in the process.

Many of Eddie's past and present colleagues, agents, friends, and teammates generously allowed me to interview them or provided background and factual content. In no particular order: Ronnie Salcer, Rick Curran, Bill Watters, Dominic Porro, David "Kap" Kaplan, Mike Lange, Bob "Hollywood" Heyden, Michael Sheehan, Mike "Doc" Emrick, Laffit Pincay III, Sam Flood, Bob Pulford, Lou Vairo, Darren "Double D" Dunn, Bob Baffert, Mike Mattine, Bob Stellick, Gord Stellick, Gary Leeman, Mark Osborne, Lorne Molleken, Rico Fata, Craig Patrick, Brian Higgins, Troy Murray, Mike Gartner, Glenn Healy, Greg Gilbert, Nick Kypreos, John Paddock, and Ray Ferraro.

I'm sure somewhere in heaven Harold Ballard and John Brophy will get a charge out of this book.

Thanks to the Chicago Blackhawks' Adam Rogowin, the Toronto Maple Leafs' Steve Keogh, the Buffalo Sabres' Chris Bandura, and the Kitchener Rangers' Treena Hennessey for their support.

And a general all-around thank-you to Jim Tatti, Norris McDonald, Jaime Macdonald, George Williams, and Ed Sousa for being great friends and advisors.

Thank you to Maury and Donna Ezra for being great friends to me and my wife, Jane.

A special thank-you to Steve Pecar, who participated in two road trips to Chicago. He's a great chauffeur and a great friend. His buddy, Joe Vecchio, provided lodging and hospitality in Detroit for me and Steve.

Thanks to Andrew Mann and Clive Farrington for "The Promise."

Thanks also to my parents, Lou and Myrna; my brother, Elliott; and my sister, Robyn, who is my guiding light.

And thanks to my in-laws, Don and Louise Lloyd.

If I have left anybody out, it was not by design or intention.

—Perry Lefko